Press & Praise for *Run Like a Girl*

"A chicken soup for the athlete's soul."
—*SELF* magazine, March 2011

"There are lots of good sports books, but rarely beautifully written
ones. *Run Like A Girl* is both."
—Mary Brophy Marcus, *USA Today*

" . . . inspiring . . . "
—*Running Times*, March 2011

"An enthusiastic tribute to women who replace the
stigma attached to the term 'running like a girl'
with a sense of power and honor."
—Kirkus Reviews

"[A] compelling argument that women who run are much more
likely to lead fulfilling lives in any number of ways . . . "
—*Canadian Running*, April 2011

"[A]n engaging read that will have most women nodding their
heads in agreement and motivated to keep at
the sports they love."
—*Vermont Sports*, April 2011

"*Run Like a Girl* celebrates the power of sports and fitness
in all aspects of life. It speaks to the true gift and value
of sport—defining who we are."
**—Julie Foudy, former Captain of the U.S.
Women's Soccer Team and founder of the
Julie Foudy Sports Leadership Academy**

"Run Like a Girl: How Strong Women Make Happy Lives strikes a chord and illustrates the transformative power of sports for women and girls. Sports enlighten, shape, and strengthen us, oftentimes enabling us to live the life we have always dreamed of. Thank you, Mina, for your commitment to documenting these stories and lessons."
—Laura Gentile, Vice President of espnW and ESPN RISE

Blogs

"A must-read for any gal athlete or aspiring gal athlete! This book will move and inspire you!"
—Marci, Triathlete4Life

"Like an encouraging voice at the toughest stretch of a race, Samuels offers the kind of support that we all crave."
—Laura Pappano, FairGameNews.com

"When simplicity and complexity reside in one sentence, I'm hooked . . . an interesting, smartly written look at the role athletics plays in the lives of women."
—Amy Moritz, Byline to Finish Line

"[J]e l'ai dévoré . . . c'est le type de livre où l'on voudra corner des pages, souligner des passages, réfléchir . . . "
/translation: " . . . I devoured it . . . it's the kind of book where you want to turn down the corners of the page, underline passages, and think . . . "
—Patrice Tessier, Mieux Vaut Courrir

Run Like a Girl

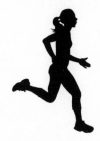

How Strong Women Make Happy Lives

Mina Samuels

SEAL PRESS

Run Like A Girl
How Strong Women Make Happy Lives

Copyright © 2011 by Mina Samuels

Published by
Seal Press
A Member of the Perseus Books Group
1700 Fourth Street
Berkeley, California

Library of Congress Cataloging-in-Publication Data

Samuels, Mina.
  Run like a girl, how strong women make happy lives / by Mina Samuels.
    p. cm.
  ISBN 978-1-58005-345-7
  1. Sports for women. 2. Sports for women--Social aspects. 3. Femininity.
I. Title.
  GV709.S35 2011
  796.082--dc22

                                        2010034054

9 8 7 6 5

Front cover image: © Ace_Create/istockphoto.com
Interior design by Tabitha Lahr
Printed in the United States of America
Distributed by Publishers Group West

To my two strong grandmothers

Clara & Lisabel

The dream is the truth.

—Zora Neale Hurston

Note

All the stories in this book are true.
Each of the women represented is an individual, never a composite.
In some cases, names have been changed to preserve privacy.

Contents

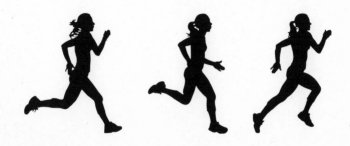

Introduction

"People don't come preassembled, but are glued together by life."
—Joseph LeDoux, neuroscientist

This book is about women, sports, and happiness. How the confidence women build in sports translates into the rest of their lives. How the challenges they face by participating in a sport, and the way they meet those challenges, translates into greater strength and the ability to overcome the obstacles in their lives outside of sports; and how their achievements in sports translate into happy lives.

This is a book about the courage it takes to challenge ourselves in how we live our lives. In the words of French philosopher and writer, Andre Gide, "[Wo]man cannot discover new oceans unless [s]he has the courage to lose sight of the shore." This is a book about many, many women who have lost sight of the shore, and found it again.

So who am I to write this book? I'm all of you, an "ordinary" woman who finds her inspiration in the stories of how other ordinary women face this ultimate challenge we call life, and perform the extraordinary feat of making it special. This is a book about women inspiring each other. Breathing in, inspiring, each other's stories. I am the lucky scribe, recording the countless stories I've been privy to over the past months as I prepared to write this book. Of course, I have my own story to add to the mix.

I discovered serious running at age twenty-seven and now participate in road races, marathons, and triathlons. I also hike, kayak, climb, do yoga, cross-country ski, and snowshoe; and as many other things as I can that get me outside in the fresh air, sun, rain, wind, and snow.

Over the years that followed my "discovery" of running, my self-confidence grew, and feeding off the accomplishments I achieved in sports—setting new personal bests, winning a little local race, surviving the setbacks of injuries and marathons gone wrong—I discovered a capacity within myself that I never knew I had. I wasn't just physically stronger than I expected, I thought of myself as a different person, as someone with more potential, broader horizons, bigger possibilities. I saw that I could push myself and take risks, not just in sports, but elsewhere, too. The competition in sports, as in life, was not with someone else, it was with myself. To "compete" was to discover my own potential to do better, to hold my own self to a higher standard, to expect more of myself—and deliver.

As William James, the nineteenth-century American philosopher, said, "Human beings, by changing the inner beliefs of their minds, can change the outer aspects of their lives."

More important than the athletic transformation I underwent was the fact that the rest of my life changed, too. I left the practice of law, charting a new course in my career—you are reading the fruit of that new career right now.

Maybe you are thinking, "What Mina just described doesn't sound so ordinary." True. And not true. Look at it this way: less than half of all Americans exercise regularly. If you cycle, or play tennis, or swim, or do yoga three or four times a week, you're not "ordinary." Of course, even if you don't do any activities with regularity, chances are there is some other aspect of your life in which you are not "ordinary" either, but as this is a book about the impact of sports on our lives, I'll stick with that, though you may find that much of what you read here is as applicable to broader pursuits as sports.

Whether you are trying to improve your own personal best or beat a worthy competitor. If you set goals, if you challenge yourself in the sports you do (and in the other things you do)—even (probably, especially) if you sometimes don't achieve what you set out to accomplish—you're not ordinary.

So what do I mean when I call myself ordinary, or indeed, when I think of the many women whose stories you'll read here as ordinary? I am not a professional athlete. Nor, indeed, are any of the women I interviewed, with a few obvious exceptions. When I meet a goal I've set in sports nothing outward changes in my life. I don't get product endorsements or coaching contracts or high-paid speaking engagements. I fit my sports in around my work and other obligations. Sometimes staying committed to the sports is an enormous struggle and I think, "I can't wait until I'm too old for this." At other times it is pure bliss and I know that I will be doing some sport for as long as I'm here. So it is for most of us.

For more than a decade, for example, racing was important to me. It's not anymore. I still race occasionally, but races are not the driving factor behind my sports, quite the contrary. I've discovered I don't need the races to motivate me and there are enough other aspects of my life where I get to be sweaty-palmed and race-nervous, like writing this book and putting it out into the world for all of you to read.

I work hard. I succeed. I fail. I have finished last more than once in a race, and at other times I've had to drop out. I try again. Sports helped me to discover that I was capable of having bigger dreams. I didn't just get fitter and faster; I changed my life. It wasn't easy. It was better than easy—it was possible and rewarding.

I need inspiration from others to keep going. And that's what this book is about—finding the inspiration to keep challenging ourselves to do better, in both our sports and our lives. I have found it in spades in all your stories.

It took a long time for me to build this writing life I wanted, and it's still a work-in-progress, as are all our lives, but at each step of the way, the accomplishment I felt in my athletic life bubbled over into the rest of my life, giving me the patience, persistence, and strength I needed to forge the path I wanted.

I'm not alone in this experience. Here are the stories and experiences of women involved in sports at every level: recreational, amateur, and, in some cases, professional; and how their involvement in sports has changed their lives for the better. Here are the climbers, the backcountry skiers, the rowers, the runners, the yoginis, the cyclists, the swimmers, the skaters, the snowshoers, the mushers, and more.

One thing connects all of our stories: to be strong in body is to be strong in mind. A woman's physical strength cannot help but become psychological strength. Strong women make happy lives.

CHAPTER 1

Do You Run Like a Girl?

"Womanhood—that takes guts."

—Shawn Hubler, columnist for the *Los Angeles Times*

What *is* running like a girl, anyway? It's getting out there. Challenging ourselves. Finding new possibility within. Finding strength in our own accomplishments. It's accessing our ageless girl spirit, where the enthusiastic "let's go" of youth meets the "I can" of experience.

Sounds great! Sign me up.

So why don't we all run like girls, all the time?

TUNING OUT RADIO KFKD

To answer that, the first place we should look is inside our heads. Here we'll find the ever-knotty true source of a woman's self-esteem.

How we feel about ourselves can run the gamut from "I suck" to "I'm so much more awesome than anyone knows!" In theory, we should fall somewhere in between self-loathing and self-aggrandizement, depending on the day. In reality, it seems like a lot of us women fall a little lower on the self-esteem scale than we should. Why? Well for one, there are myriad voices, those of our culture and our peers—but especially our own—that insinuate themselves into our head, feeding us nonsense about everything from our appearance and self-worth to our strength and capabilities.

Sexy is a Victoria's Secret model and that's sooooo not you, with your frizzy hair and plum-size breasts.

What is that, you're thinking of getting a master's degree? Who are you kidding, there's no way you could finish an entire thesis.

And now you're thinking of running a marathon? Yeah, right! You've never run farther than three miles in a stretch.

Ouch!

Worse, the trash-talking voices that invade our psyche are downright villainous in their power to gut our confidence and prevent us from living a fully realized life, one we're *capable* of living, as strong women, running like girls.

I should know. My head is *filled* with trash talk. . . .

When I was young, my parents were adherents of the well-worn proverb "pride cometh before a fall." I constantly worried that too much self-confidence might become pride, and that would be a *bad* thing. I lived with the fear that any budding sense of achievement I might feel was on a dangerous, slippery slope to being "too big for my britches" or becoming someone with a "swelled head." Not surprisingly, I had trouble finding and maintaining a healthy sense of self-confidence. I've since come to realize that my parents must have left off a key first word to the proverb: excessive.

Yet to this day if someone says to me, "You must be proud of . . ." anything from a marathon time to a work-related project, I feel myself physically shy away from the inference. Me? Proud? No way.

So where is that line between prideful and not? And who dictates where the line is drawn anyway? Are confidence and pride just the same thing looked at from different angles?

Maybe you're one of the lucky few who escaped the female epidemic of devaluing and underestimating ourselves.

I am not.

Nor are most of the women who shared their stories for this book. And yet, in the realm of sports, our tendency to minimize our accomplishments, even put ourselves down, can't stand up to the scrutiny of our athletic accomplishments. Sports take determination and strength, making it hard to denigrate our abilities. Sports are quantitative proof of our capacity.

At the turn of the twentieth century, in a speech titled "The Outlook of Gymnastics" at Newcomb College's symposium on physical culture, student Leila Green said, "It was so interesting, you know, so really aristocratic, to be an invalid; and dear me, it was once actually quite vulgar to be well and robust and altogether healthy."

 "'[I]t was once actually quite vulgar to be well and robust and altogether healthy.'"

Unfortunately, Leila's message was a little ahead of its time. Almost a century later, sports were still considered a vulgar pastime for some women.

When Michelle Theall, the former editor-in-chief of *Women's Adventure Magazine*, was growing up, her parents encouraged her to quit sports because her mother "didn't see the value."

When Sarah Armstrong played rugby in college, her parents were less than enthusiastic. "They hated this unladylike pastime of mine and taunted me incessantly," she says.

Well none of that is going to help a growing girl's self-esteem. Letting our battered confidence diminish our capacities is just another form of being that aristocratic invalid Leila Green mentioned so long ago. But that's not all. Instead of feeling empowered by society to revel in our vulgar strength, we often feel it's almost our duty as women to be self-deprecating instead of self-affirming.

Consider this: how much time does it take for two women who have just met to express their mutual self-doubts or enumerate their shortcomings?

Answer: no time at all.

When you meet another woman, do you begin by sharing your accomplishments? I'm not even talking about the pissing matches men can get into, of who's caught the biggest fish (metaphorical or real). Or do you ease into the new friendship by commiserating about how your hair is too thin or too frizzy, or your

"When you meet another woman, do you begin by sharing your accomplishments?"

butt is too flat or too big, or you have too many freckles. Too often we bond through belittling ourselves, feeding our low self-esteem, as if deflating our confidence is something worthwhile. What's that about?

Anne Lamott had a great answer. In her classic book *Bird by Bird*, she writes about our internal radio station, which you can find on the dial at Radio KFKD, and yes, it is how it sounds, a nonstop station playing too much trash. One minute those internal airwaves tell us we're great and the next minute the message is that we're worthless and should just give up.

Let's turn the dial down. In fact—let's turn K-Fucked *off*. The world might seem a mite quiet at first, but don't worry, that's just the sound of courage.

As Shawn Hubler, a columnist for the *Los Angeles Times*, wrote, "It isn't an easy thing for a girl to grow up to be a woman, not nearly as easy as it is for her to grow up to remain a girl. You can spend a lifetime in this world acting winsome and blaming your troubles on PMS and men. But womanhood—that takes guts."

TRAILBLAZING IS NOT FOR THE WINSOME

I read an illuminating piece by business blogger Whitney Johnson on the Harvard Business Publishing website. Apparently, women who negotiate for higher salaries generally don't get the same pay increase as their male counterparts. That's not necessarily breaking news. What is worth noting, however, is the fact that they are actually *frowned* upon for having asked. It's an insidious way of discouraging us further from pursuing our due because it plays upon our desire to be liked, to be part of the team. After all, nice girls don't ask for pay rises, or actually much of anything. So we're in a double bind—if you don't ask, you won't get it; if you do ask, you're a pushy bitch. What interested me most about the post was Johnson's point that we women must keep asking, even if people don't perceive us as "nice." And that by asking, we are not only standing up for ourselves, we are standing up for *all* women.

When we set precedents in the world as strong women, as women with guts—whether it's asking for pay raises or climbing mountains, literally—we smooth the path, pave the way, lay the groundwork, so to speak, for the girls who are coming up behind us. How cool is that? In case you thought your risk-taking and accomplishments weren't important, think again.

 "In case you thought your risk-taking and accomplishments weren't important, think again."

Yet when we trail blaze, men are not the only ones who might think we're not being "nice."

In 1991, professional tennis player Monica Seles publicly stated that tournament prize money should be equal for men and women. Not only did she *not* succeed in achieving parity between the purses awarded to each gender, but other women tennis players sided against Seles and were quoted as saying things like, "We don't need more," and "I don't think we should be greedy." I wonder if those women tennis players are giving back their extra "greedy" money, because thanks to efforts like Seles's, tennis purses are closer to equal than in any other sport.

Too often, being a trailblazer for other women isn't always greeted with enthusiasm or acceptance. Gayle Barron, who won the Boston Marathon for women in 1978, once said that she struggled with being a pioneer. Not so much because of men's attitudes, but because her women friends thought she ought to be at home with her family, in "a woman's place." Her friends didn't celebrate her successes. Worse still, they disapproved. She wonders how much she held back from achieving her true potential for the sake of keeping her friends.

Things have changed. Certainly Serena and Venus Williams aren't going to play shy when it comes to getting what they want on the tennis court. Nor does it seem likely that Paula Radcliffe or Kara Goucher's friends will get on their cases for prioritizing their blazing running careers. We can thank Monica and Gayle and all the many other trailblazers for the privilege of enjoying our strength unimpeded. Fewer and fewer women are willing to sit quietly under the falling shards of broken glass ceilings, in sports or anywhere else. When we aren't holding ourselves or other women back, there is so much we can be and do.

Joelle Schmitz, a downhill skier and senior fellow at Harvard's Mossavar-Rahmani Center for Business and Government, says she definitely feels her responsibility to the girls who will come next.

When she was climbing Tuckerman's Ravine (widely considered to be one of the most dangerous hike-up and ski-down mountains in the United States), she was keenly conscious of the men hundreds of feet below her, "and of their pathetic determination to avoid getting 'chicked.'" That is, to be beaten up the mountain by a woman. "I think of the metaphor of preteen cheerleaders socialized to objectify themselves rather than assume a place next to the boys in the field," says Joelle. "I think of the little girls who watch me intently as I beat their fathers over the Giant Slalom finish line. . . . I have a responsibility to manifest."

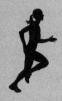 **"'I think of the little girls who watch me intently as I beat their fathers over the Giant Slalom finish line. . . . I have a responsibility to manifest.'"**

We can all take on that responsibility; after all, the obligation doesn't weigh much. Quite the opposite. Blazing trails, as Joelle so vividly demonstrates, can be exhilarating. As can running like a girl.

WOMEN ARE NOT SMALL MEN

Doing research for this book, I learned a new sports retail term—"shrinking and pinking." The expression refers to how athletic clothing and gear were (and still are in some cases) designed to accommodate women. Manufacturers would "shrink" men's clothing and gear down to women's sizes—without consideration of the differences in our physiology, kinetics, shape, and ability—then offer the shrunken product in pink. I learned the term from Kim Walker, the founder of Outdoor Divas, a women's clothing and gear store based in Colorado. For her, the business was a result of Plato's ancient truism: necessity is the mother of invention.

Inspiration came after Kim finished college, when she and her boyfriend moved to Vail to be ski bums for a while.

"I didn't actually ski that well, but he did, so he taught me," Kim says. She'd arrive at the top of snowy mountains sporting long, straight skis she couldn't maneuver with her smaller frame, then clumsily follow a bunch of men down too-steep terrain. "I was frustrated a lot," she says, having to muscle her way through every learning experience. The same pattern replayed itself for kayaking, rock climbing, and mountain biking. She learned by being thrown into situations in which she was out of her depth, with the added bonus of bad equipment that didn't account for the physical differences between men and women.

Not surprisingly, many women abandon sports after an experience like Kim's. They have no idea that what seemed to be outside their capacity is really only the limitations of poorly designed equipment and training, but they don't stick around long enough to find out. Part of the problem is that role models are sparse, particularly in what have traditionally been the more "macho" sports, like mountain biking and rock climbing. If our mothers and aunts and the girl next door aren't doing the sports, it can be hard to find the models in the media.

As Heidi Van Es, a marathoner and social worker from New York, asks, "Who's on the front page of the sports section? Predominantly men."

Lois Harrison, a flight attendant and runner in her sixties, says sports were all about men when she was growing up in the 1950s. And despite the gains women have made—including better news coverage—even now when she plays tennis with a girlfriend, she says that the men playing on adjacent courts act as if she and her tennis partner are not there, even walking through their court to get stray balls.

A girl thinking about becoming an athlete is going to have to dig deeper than the sports section to find her role models.

 "A girl thinking about becoming an athlete is going to have to dig deeper than the sports section to find her role models."

In her own life, Heidi was lucky. At her high school, the physical education instructors who were women were strong and beautiful. They would run with the girls three times a week. The male instructors, on the other hand, were fat and out of shape and couldn't have run with the girls if they'd wanted to. So from early on, Heidi had models of strong women. She knew that sports were worth her time and effort.

As athletes, we can be powerful role models both on and off the field—or, as in Kristy's case, off the rink. Kristy Powell, who plays ice hockey and is on the U.S. Women's Bandy Team, has been playing hockey since she was five years old, almost thirty years now. As you can imagine, this is *not* the most welcoming sport for girls or women. Boys have made obscene noises at her on the ice. Once, she says, she was even encouraged to tuck her ponytail into her shoulder pads so the other team wouldn't notice she was a girl. In other words, just to lace up the skates and get on the ice took moxie.

One day, she was in Sports Authority picking up some new hockey equipment when a girl around eight years old picked out a pair of pink hockey gloves. With a big smile she showed them to her mother, "Look at these cool gloves, Mom. Can I play hockey?" The excitement and hope in the young girl's voice was palpable, Kristy says. The mother said, "Girls don't play hockey. It's not feminine."

Kristy was stunned and not a little frustrated. She picked up the pink hockey mouth guard she had been looking for, and then she couldn't help herself, she walked over to the mother and daughter and asked politely, "Excuse me, but I wonder if I could ask you a question? Do you think that I'm feminine?" She was wearing a skirt, and her pixie haircut, with fashionable blond tips, could hardly be called masculine. The mother, somewhat taken aback by Kristy's directness, answered, "Feminine, I guess."

Kristy thanked her, looked at the young girl, and told her about how she was picking up a pink mouth guard in preparation to go skate professionally in Sweden. Then she said, "Girls can play any sport they want and maintain their femininity. It's all in how you were raised."

Or not, because despite early discouragement and boy equipment, even if it has been shrinked and pinked, we can prevail. Outdoor Diva Kim stuck with her sports and she's now an expert skier (not to mention kayaker, mountain biker, and climber). She also stuck with the boyfriend, who is now her husband and father of their son. And what do you know, *together* they recognized there was a niche to be filled for the countless women frustrated by their boyfriend's hand-me-downs, and they founded Outdoor Divas.

"Everyone told us we were crazy," says Kim. "People said it was folly to split the market, that women didn't want their own place to shop."

Really? If such a store existed in New York City, I guess I'd only shop there 95 percent of the time.

"If you have a really great idea, run with it," says Kim. "Take advice and constructive criticism from experts, but never let them quash your dream."

Their company slogan?—Women are not small men.

WHERE THE GIRLS ARE . . . ON THEIR OWN

Male-dominated sports pages, shrinked and pinked sporting goods stores—sometimes it's nice to escape what can seem like a pretty androcentric sports world. Not only in North America, but throughout the world, women *own* their bodies and feel freer to learn and test their abilities when they do sports together, free of men.

That's where participating in all-women training camps come in. They can be a welcome relief and a big confidence builder. We don't have to compete with the gender naturally endowed with more physical strength. They are free of men who think they should automatically be faster or stronger than the women (even if, poor boys, they aren't always). The experience rarely starts with participants exchanging puffed-up sports accomplishments. And the pressure to perform is mostly relieved. Instead, it's replaced by an environment of support and encouragement. At a women's mountain biking clinic I once went to, we more often found ourselves psyching each other up at the top of a steep descent instead of daring each other to shred down the hill without regard for life and limb. And there was no shame in walking our bikes if the terrain just didn't feel forgiving. For me, paradoxically, this low-stress environment is exactly what I need to build confidence and ultimately perform better. "You can do it," is miles more helpful than "This is nothing. You should have seen what I rode last week." Not that we were not competitive in the clinic. We were. But with ourselves. To end better than we had started, that was the only goal.

Even my earliest memories of feeling truly independent and strong are rooted in my experiences of going to an all-girl's summer camp when I was young. Those summers furnished me with some of my earliest memories of feeling comfortable in my skin. Unburdened by the teen anxiety of whether I was of interest to the boys, I could be myself. I could leave off worrying about why everyone else had breasts, while mine were only hinting at existence. I didn't feel like

"Unburdened by the teen anxiety of whether I was of interest to the boys, I could be myself."

I had to wrestle my hair into an acceptable approximation of Farrah Fawcett's feathered look. There were no points to be gained for being pretty and pulled together, for being demure. Instead, I could devote all my energy to the activities I loved—canoeing, swimming, orienteering, and the camp musical. I could be rough and ready without feeling frowned on for being a tomboy. I wonder, too, how much of the physical strength I learned to own at summer camp translated into my good grades in school. More than I thought, I'll bet.

A cross-sectional study by the California Department of Education found that girls demonstrated higher academic achievement at higher fitness levels than did boys. And a study by the

Centers for Disease Control and Prevention found that time spent in "phys ed" may improve a girl's academic performance, while it made no change in a boy's.

Here's a microcosm of that statistic: Lisa Leshne, a literary agent and marathoner in her forties, went to a small high school in the Midwest during the mid-1980s. The top three students in the school were all girls, and what's more, they were all top athletes—state champions in running, swimming, and basketball.

One last small interesting fact—if universities accepted strictly on academic achievement, with no eye to gender balance, at least 60 percent of university students would be women. And the women's sports teams would be as good as ever.

No wonder some women may get obsessed by having it all—it turns out we're well equipped to have it all.

And we North American women are lucky. We face only a fraction of the obstacles faced by women elsewhere in the world.

Sarah Murray, who worked for the Women's Sports Foundation and is accomplished in many sports, took a time-out in her career to travel around the world. One of the many fascinating things she learned during her trip was the difference between sports in a woman's life in the United States versus the role of sports in the developing countries she traveled through. Here, the sports women pursue are just one aspect of a largely independent life. Though sports here can be a cornerstone of a woman's sense of self, without sports there are still plenty of opportunities for us to explore our potential.

In Africa and South Asia, however, the relevance of sports cut closer to the bone; the impact is deeper and often more singular. Sports are the lifeblood for girls and women involved in them—whether it is the Ethiopian runners, the South African soccer players, or the Nepalese trekkers that Sarah met.

"The sports these women were involved in were often the only time they *owned* their bodies," Sarah says. When they aren't on the field or trail, societal norms clamp down on their lives.

 "'The sports these women were involved in were often the only time they *owned* their bodies.'"

Their roles and responsibilities as caregivers for their families, from a very young age, and then as mothers (often very young, too), afford them no opportunity to explore their own needs and desires. Their bodies are for birthing and chores. That is, until they discover sports, or indeed something else, that shows them another possibility.

Shoe4Africa is just one organization showing women that more is possible. A nonprofit organization based in the United States and Kenya, Shoe4Africa uses sports and education to empower communities in Africa. Here's what's on their women's empowerment page:

> [T]he women of Africa are waiting in the wings, we proved it in a very small way: In Iten village, Kenya, there was a race where six women and 126 men turned up to run, the women told us, "The men tell us stay home, running is not for you . . . that is why our numbers

are so few." So we held a women's only race in that village
of 4,000 inhabitants. We had 2,900 women come to line
up! That is the Women of Africa . . . they are ready for
leadership and building stability in a continent crying to
get back to its peaceful ways.

Around the world, women find their feet, their focus, and their strength through sports. They feel *empowered*. Of course, women here didn't always enjoy such freedoms, either—in both mind and body. In 1896, Susan B. Anthony said, "Bicycling has done more to emancipate women than any one thing in the world." And Susan B. was a woman who knew about taking risks. Thanks to her and many other suffragists' willingness to do jail time, we women have the right to vote. I like voting and cycling, so I count myself lucky to live in a time and place where I can do both.

Our emancipation was only getting started with the vote, it turns out; since then there have been a host of laws that have enhanced our opportunities and unbound us from society's strictures (thank you Roe v. Wade), bringing us ever closer to the full breadth of possibility. When it comes to sports, the most powerful law was Title IX.

FIRST, RUN LIKE A BOY, THEN . . .

Until Title IX passed in 1972, women had to fight to run like girls, not to mention ski, climb, swim, row, cycle, and dunk, to name only a few. The law, an education amendment that was phased in over time, mandates equality between girls and boys in school-based sports. And there is no denying its impact.

According to the National Federation of State High School Associations, between the school years 1970–71 and 1977–78, girls' participation in sports increased 600 percent. That's a lot of girls lacing up their cleats and skates, and putting on their first sports bra. I like to imagine a mass of ponytailed girls converging on to fields and into gymnasiums, temporarily sidelining a bunch of gawky young boys flummoxed by the sudden estrogen invasion.

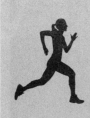

"[I]magine a mass of ponytailed girls converging on to fields and into gymnasiums, temporarily sidelining a bunch of gawky young boys flummoxed by the sudden estrogen invasion."

Recent studies have also found that Title IX has been enormously positive beyond just increasing participation. In a 2010 report titled "Beyond the Classroom: Using Title IX to Measure the Return to High School Sports," Wharton School economist Betsey Stevenson outlines a study she conducted linking participation in high school sports to a girl's achievement later in life. Stevenson's study, published by the National Bureau of Economic Research, showed a direct relationship between Title IX, the increase in women's education, and the overall rise in women's employment. She found that nearly 40 percent of the increase in employment among 25- to 34-year-old women could be tied to their experiences playing sports.

"Sports help people do better in life," says Stevenson. And with statistics showing that tens of millions of girls have taken up the opportunity to play sports in high school in the thirty years since Title IX was fully implemented, that's a lot of empowerment. In fact, Stevenson found that playing sports leads not only to greater female participation in the workforce but largely in previously male-dominated, high-skill careers. There's a reason why the title "doctor" can no longer be assumed to mean "mister."

Other research has shown links between girls' participation in sports and lower teen pregnancy rates, better grades, higher self-esteem, lower obesity rates, and better health as an adult. Literally running *as* a girl has a profound impact on her future as a woman.

So, Title IX has clearly had deep effects. But our work is not done. There are still cases of disparity, particularly when it comes to role models for these increasing numbers of girls entering sports. Strangely, for example, there's been a decrease in the number of women hired as physical education teachers, an unfortunate trend at a time when we hope for more role models, not less.

Equality in sports is a work in progress. The efforts toward equality have been going on for some time, possibly since the Greek goddess Artemis picked up her bow, and will for some time more.

Given our milestones toward equality, sometimes we assume women's rights are an "old" issue. But consider this: The women's marathon was not an official Olympic event until 1984. To get the event sanctioned required medical certification that marathons were not harmful to women, that women were indeed strong enough to do the distance. Wow, 1984. That's hardly ancient history.

To this day, there still remain Olympic sports that do not include women. Ski jumping is the lone male-only sport in the Winter Olympic Games. The original reason women weren't allowed to participate in the sport was the belief that, like with marathon running, it was somehow medically deleterious to the female body; something about jarring "the female organism," whatever that means. I suppose I should be grateful that the International Olympic Committee (IOC) is so concerned about women's health. Yet I can't help but think that women should have the right to decide what's healthy for them or not when it comes to aggressive sports. And even though women have since received a doctor's note saying it's alright to participate, the IOC now argues that they haven't opened the competition to women because the field of women ski jumpers isn't deep enough, which seems a thin reason given that it's likely not any deeper in the new Olympic sport of ski cross, or even ice hockey, which are both open to women.

Annette Hofmann, a professor of sports studies at the Ludwigsburg University of Education in Germany, believes that the real reason women aren't being included is that they may soon jump farther than men. The winning jumpers these days are anorexic men, since the sport favors lean and small. Prior to the 2010 Winter Games, the record holder on the Olympic jump at Whistler was a woman, Lindsey Van. Hofmann speculates that the participation of women in the sport would threaten the "virile image" of the sport. As in, we will have no flying pink ski suits.

The power of liberating laws like Title IX, even the near-parity in Olympic sports (they can't keep us out of ski jumping for much longer), may not always be enough to open our horizons, to take our rightful place beside men, off the sidelines. Remember those insidious little voices? And the naysayers who didn't want to be paid more for playing tennis?—well they are all part and parcel of our own conditioning about gender expectations. Turns out we are quite adept at getting in our own way.

Molly Barker, the founder of Girls on the Run, was walking home from a work meeting not too long ago, dressed in a skirt. Coming toward her on the sidewalk was a group of men in business suits. Without waiting to see what they might do, she moved aside and walked around them. Sometime later that same day, as she was heading out on her run, she ran into the same group of suited men. Except *this* time she ran right through the middle of them.

Why? What had changed? As strong and independent as Molly is, there are still times when she feels like a bit of an object under the eyes of men, as when she's in her skirt, in her conventional female disguise. But once she's laced up her running shoes, she says there's no oxygen left for that feeling. "Whatever those men might be thinking, I no longer feel them looking at me as an object. I'm free."

 "'Whatever those men might be thinking, I no longer feel them looking at me as an object. I'm free.'"

We all want to carry that sense of freedom to be exactly who we are into every corner of our lives. The unfortunate truth is that it can be hard. Even Molly, who has dedicated her life to helping girls understand how the strength they feel from running enables them to expand so much more in the rest of their lives, struggles at times. If feeling free to be as strong as we want were not a challenge, we might forget. We might forget what we're running for, what we've gained and all that's possible.

For girls in particular, sports are one of the most important ways in which we can be empowered. Or so believes Mary Wittenberg, president and CEO of New York Road Runners. Through sports, as Mary points out, we learn that to run like a girl we need to also run like a stereotypical boy—to seize opportunity, to challenge ourselves, to test ourselves, to jump in with both feet, to believe in our ability—all the things that boys have taken for granted for so long, but that have traditionally come harder to our fairer sex.

What we bring, as girls, to running like a boy is our ability to take things step by step—to be more thoughtful about our goals, to build slowly toward them; not necessarily start with a marathon, but start with a mile. Achieve and set a higher ambition. Achieve that next level and set another higher ambition. Or not. We could just jump in and start with something big, whatever moves you. There isn't just one way to run like a girl, because RLAG (running like a girl) is about possibility. And possibility is inclusive, of each other and the choices we make.

THE POWER OF "FEMININE"

When I interviewed Kathrine Switzer, the first woman to legally run the Boston Marathon in 1967, we talked some feminism, no surprise given her resume. In addition to that first Boston, it includes a long list of efforts on behalf of women in sports, including the campaign to get the women's marathon approved by the IOC, and starting a nationwide series of women's races.

When I use the term "feminism," I mean it in the broadest, most inclusive "third-wave" sense, as women who define, own, and express their needs, desires, strength, and independence, and have the liberty and right to do so in the way they see fit. But let's back up for a moment. "First-wave" feminism is generally considered the women's suffrage movement, gaining the political right to vote. "Second-wave" feminism is then defined as the civil and cultural rights, like equal pay, reproductive freedom, and equal opportunity, like Title IX. By the 1990s, however, there was a sense that the first two waves did not adequately address the issues faced by women of diverse ethnicities, nationalities, religions, and cultural backgrounds; thus, the third wave, which recognized that there could be no single feminist ideal. Just as there is no single ideal woman.

From the beginning, Kathrine dedicated herself to getting women into sports and sports into women, so she faced a lot of opposition. Men would often ask her the following question, both rhetorical and not: "What's up with you women and running?"

"Men would often ask her the following question, both rhetorical and not: 'What's up with you women and running?'"

Some women who consider themselves feminists might walk away from a question that feels so hostile, or even meet the query with defensiveness. I know I might be very tempted to fight fire with fire. Not Kathrine. She would sit down and talk to those men. Explain what's up with women and running. After all, what's the goal? A battle or to share the gift of running (or any other sport) with as many women as possible; which, when Kathrine first began promoting women's rights, was only going to happen when men were on board, too. Kathrine's gift early on was to see that alternative and use it to all our advantage. She's not the first or last person to understand the wisdom of this mind-set, but she is a living example of compassion in action.

As we're on the topic of feminism, now is a good time for a story from a woman who learned how to run like a girl—well, actually *throw* and *hit* like a girl, and this before the term feminism was coined.

Claire McPherson, who founded the first dance therapy program in the United States, started playing handball when she was around ten years old, in 1938. "I was a very active child," she says, "all I was told was to sit still."

But she couldn't. She took dance classes in the afterschool Yiddish program, but then her parents curtailed that because they didn't see the point of dance. So Claire took herself off to the playground and started playing handball.

For the uninitiated, handball is an outdoor street game that is played, for the most part, in school playgrounds. To get on the court (at least in Claire's era), she had to wait on the sidelines until one of the boys tired and dropped out and no boys remained to replace him. As a girl, Claire had to establish and re-establish her ability to play, to be accepted into the handball games. She still remembers the feeling of outrage she experienced standing on the sidelines, having to prove herself to even get on the court.

"I'm as good as half of those boys, even better than some, and they're not letting me play," she'd think. Because she was good at handball, she got off the sidelines, but that sense of outrage politicized Claire. Long before the women's movement had gathered steam, much less feminism, Claire had fought and earned her independence in sports.

"Playing handball is a sport where you use yourself fully, something women didn't often have the opportunity to do," Claire says. "You have to be quick, direct, and strong."

Traits that Claire's friends and colleagues would use to describe her off the playground, too.

This became clear when Claire joined her first women's consciousness group in the late 1960s. She quickly realized she wasn't facing the same issues as most of the other women in her group. They were wondering how to get out of the house. She was out of the house. They were struggling to find balance and equality in their marriages. Claire had established that dynamic with her husband, whom she'd met on a basketball court, from the outset.

"But I *could* teach them how to throw a ball," she says. And she did.

Claire taught them how to "throw from the bottom of their toes." And the women felt good about themselves in a whole new way. They discovered what they weren't "using" of themselves. They learned how to "maximize" themselves to accomplish the goal of throwing well.

"Claire taught them how to 'throw from the bottom of their toes.' And the women felt good about themselves in a whole new way."

When we learn what it feels like to be inside our skin, to pull from the deep well of our inner resources, to maximize ourselves in one area, it is much easier to bring that knowledge to bear everywhere else in our lives.

Now in her early eighties, Claire is still going strong. She teaches a course on dreams to seniors, and she does Pilates.

"Women don't need to call themselves feminists anymore," Claire says.

We can simply live as feminists.

FEEL THE WIND BENEATH YOUR SKIRT

As with feminism, running like a girl needs to be inclusive of the broadest range of women. So you want to run? Great. You don't also have to be the worn-out stereotype of a tomboy. You can wear pink. Or you can wear black. Sparkles and bows, or slouch jeans and a ripped T-shirt.

We know all this about having the biggest tent possible, and yet too often we can be guilty of judging other women as "not feminist enough," either because of behavior, dress, or lifestyle. I know I've caught myself shrinking the tent. How about this one: How can a woman take the sport of running seriously if she's wearing a skirt? Guilty as charged. That's me, thinking, *Does she need to look so girly?* I thought, *Skirts are fluffy; running shouldn't be.* I thought, *If we women want to be taken seriously, then we should wear serious running clothes.*

And yet, how does running make us feel? Answer: strong, capable, powerful, and yes, here it is, *sexy*. And how do short femmy skirts make us feel? Do you see where I'm going? Running and skirts don't have to be mutually exclusive.

During the expo in Saint Petersburg, Florida, for the Women's Running Magazine Half Marathon, Kathrine Switzer and I stopped by the booth of a clothing company aptly named Running Skirts. Kathrine, it turned out, was picking up a skirt that she'd ordered. I smiled politely at the two women who founded the company, pretending to be open to the whole notion. Running skirts, by the way, are literally skirts designed specifically for running. Think of them as an updated sibling to tennis skirts. The women at the booth discovered I didn't own a running skirt, and I could barely be encouraged to try one on. But I did to be polite. *Well, the skirt fit okay,* I thought, raising an internal eyebrow. But I tried to give it back nonetheless. "No, take it," they said. I promised the women, a bit halfheartedly, that I'd wear the skirt during the race the next day.

I did.

And a strange thing happened. I felt kind of cute, in a speedy way. I felt fleet and sleek, like I had a secret power, like I had hidden retro-rockets under my skirt. In other words, I felt like a strong woman.

 "I felt fleet and sleek, like I had a secret power, like I had hidden retro-rockets under my skirt."

Laura Cozik, the founder of Team Lipstick, a New York–based all-women's triathlon team, came from the world of competitive ballroom dancing where "If it didn't sparkle, why wear it?"

For her team of women who are new to triathlons, she is designing race-specific clothes with a bit more flair than the usual triathlon attire (which are designed to perform efficiently throughout the swim-bike-run). If anyone can figure out the strategic placement of a sequin on a race kit so the ornamentation won't cause abrasion during a race, Laura will. And she's getting women who haven't owned a bike since childhood, let alone swim, to complete races they thought they could never do.

"The hottest thing about a person is confidence," says Laura.

Sports give us confidence. Feeling sexy gives us confidence. Put the two together and watch out.

As Lynn Martel, a devotee of mountain sports, says, "Being competent in my activities makes me want to look like a girl even more. I detest wearing black, even to formal events. I'm much happier in emerald green or teal!"

That running skirt, even in plain old black, which I admit I'm partial to, gave me confidence. This is not an advertisement for running wear—but I have to finish the story by saying that the skirt worked its magic. I didn't do the time I wanted, but I did well, placing ninth out of 3,276 women. Of course, the skirt wasn't responsible for my race result. And yet, I couldn't help but think that the skirt *was*. The new attire was the symbolic representation of something bigger—that I had opened myself up to something new, in spite of my biases.

I turned my back on my own resistance. I owned my own strength just a little bit more. I credit Kathrine with that, too: being around her energy, her conviction, and her expansiveness, and the ownership she takes of being a woman and an athlete. By the way, she wore a cheetah print running skirt for the race. *Pow! Shazam!*

We run like girls when we run *for* ourselves and *inside* ourselves. We run like girls when we tune out the negativity that might come our way—from men, from women, from any of myriad sources, including ourselves. We run like girls when we own our power, when we celebrate what we are capable of, when we take joy from our vulgar strength.

The first time I went out solo in a canoe I felt the kind of strength and sureness that running skirt gave me.

I was fourteen, at an all-girls camp in northern Ontario called Camp Glen Bernard. I can still feel the moment as if it is written on my body. . . .

The lake is flat, whorls of fine mist across the surface. The prehistoric squawk of a heron floats across the water. In the distance I can see the great bird slowly flapping its huge wings.

In the canoe, I kneel on my lifejacket, legs folded beneath me. I settle my weight so the boat tilts enough for me to hold my paddle deep in the water for a more powerful stroke. Then I'm off, alone, pulling the canoe forward in smooth surges. I feel the muscles in my shoulders and back flex and release. Two forward pulls and a J-stroke to keep the boat straight. The boat moves fast toward the middle of the lake, where there is no one.

My mind empties. I'm watching as the water falls away from the paddle, like a stream slipping over rocks, flat cascades running sideways away from the paddle with each stroke. The color of the water shifts between green and blue. Bubbles burst from the paddle and jostle each other to the surface and then the jeweled drops slide across the surface of the paddle as I pull it from the water to end the stroke. The drops hang on the edges and tip of the paddle, momentarily suspended in defiance of gravity. And for each new diamond drop, I wonder if it will be the one that changes the laws of physics and does not detach itself to fall twinkling into the lake, to disappear among the infinite number of other drops.

Beams of sunlight penetrate only a few inches beneath the surface, capturing all the tiny algae and water insects in its rays, like watery dust motes.

I practice my canoe strokes, pulling the boat in tight circles with a C-stroke, forward then backward, watching the horizon swing by, then skulling to move the boat sideways, and cutting to turn the boat quickly. I don't think about anything except the boat and the water, the bubbles fluttering loose with each stroke, as if a pixie stood on the tip of my paddle, blowing soap through a ring.

I feel strong and sure and capable. The canoe moves effort-lessly, as if my legs have been replaced by the boat. I am a mermaid. I am magic. I am a girl on the brink of womanhood.

CHAPTER 2:

Discovering Our Magic Shoes

"How much longer will you go on letting your energy sleep?
How much longer are you going to stay oblivious
of the immensity of yourself?"
—Bhagwan Shree Rajneesh, philosopher

I didn't always run like a girl.

Sure, I had *run* before—short struggles with the sidewalk; occasional hills punctuated by moments spent gasping for oxygen. I was fit, as much as anyone else around me seemed to be. Teaching aerobics classes had helped pay for law school, and the firm I eventually worked for offered free gym memberships. Waste a perk? Not me. I'd even bumbled through a couple of triathlons. (Note to self: best to actually know how to use swim goggles prior to swimming.)

Sports were a means to an end—being reasonably healthy—not an end in themselves, not something I participated in for the sheer pleasure of the experience.

It wasn't that I was averse to exercise. I had grown up in a vigorous, outdoorsy kind of family—we went car camping and my brothers and I loved to play in the woods at my grandparents' apple farm. We often walked instead of drove, and my father cycled on the weekends, a rearview mirror attached to his helmet, carrying saddlebags filled with enough spare parts to build a whole new bicycle en route, should the need arise. For a short time, I even joined the school track and field team. From watching the Olympics, I thought crouching down in the starting blocks looked akin to being in a personal rocket launcher, and how fun would *that* be? But I gave up track when my period started, embarrassed by how maxi pads looked with my underwear-style track shorts. Plus, being athletic was definitely *not* cool for girls at my school. Later, when my youngest brother got into mountain bike racing, somehow I thought it was right that he, a *boy*, should be the one doing the more serious sport.

I retreated indoors, went to university, then work, wore suits and stockings, and ate my dinners working late at the office. The outdoors was something I mostly passed through on the way to somewhere else. From an unexceptional background I was building an ordinary life.

Was I happy? Kind of. Sort of. Well . . . not really.

IF I CAN RUN A MARATHON . . .

It all started when my friend Jacquie dropped out of the sky in the Israeli desert, narrowly missing a Bedouin.

What started as a seemingly benign adventure, a half-day parasailing lesson, ended in a shattered right heel. Her foot became a weather beacon, able to predict rain and damp with startling accuracy *and* painful swelling.

A few months later, my friend's wife, Olivia, gave birth to their first child. The baby was healthy and happy, scoring in the top percentile of every infant testing category, but Olivia failed to top the charts in her own recovery. A crippling version of postpartum diabetes rendered her wheelchair-bound within the year. Not long afterward, my upstairs neighbor, Kathleen, was stricken with an insidious rheumatoid arthritis that stiffened and puffed up her joints. She who once reveled in the sensual pleasures of cheddar, brie, and ice cream became immobilized if she indulged in anything with a whiff of dairy. On the days she didn't touch dairy, she coped with what's euphemistically called "manageable pain."

Though their health issues were different, these three women shared something in common: they had all been young, healthy, and vibrant. The future was theirs. When they had time, they were going to do the things they *really* enjoyed, like get more exercise, go on long trips, paint. For now they were building their lives. They were young and time seemed infinite.

And then it wasn't.

The tomorrow-rug was pulled right out from under them. A myriad of "would'ves" and "gonnas" fell around their feet. I *would've* run a marathon. I was *gonna* go whitewater canoeing in Canada's Northwest Territories.

"How quickly the joys of owning a body can be snatched from us," psychologist April Martin wrote in her essay "Dreams on Ice," words that resonated deeply for me when I read them, perfectly capturing the urgent feeling of physical "temporariness" I experienced as a result of these three women's health crises. Like my friends, I had a long list of adventures and achievements I thought I'd do later when I established my so-called *real* life more firmly: climb a mountain, go backpacking, travel to every continent. Run a marathon and write a novel didn't even figure on the to-do list yet. They were on the "I can only dream of that" list. I had no idea yet that to do the things I wanted, or even *dreamed* of, was only a matter of courage, the courage to believe in myself.

I had recently made one change in my life, taking an eight-month leave of absence from the law firm I worked for to pursue a Master of Laws degree, which meant moving from Toronto to New York, where I didn't know a soul. Deep in studies, confined to a typically microscopic New York apartment, I needed an occasional escape to clear my head. I started running a few days a week. At first

"Deep in studies, confined to a typically microscopic New York apartment, I needed an occasional escape to clear my head."

I ran along the perimeter of Central Park because I was too scared to actually go *into* the park alone, then finally I mustered the temerity to venture inside its walls. Surprise! There were other runners, *lots* of them. Before I knew it, I had worked up the endurance to run a whole loop of Central Park, almost ten kilometers in one shot.

One day in the law library, a woman I hoped to befriend asked me about my running. "Oh I run about ten, three times a week," I said airily. I was somewhat intimidated by her. She had run marathons, something inconceivable to me. In truth, I had only once run three times in a week, but I was determined to do it more often, so I felt only mildly guilty telling her it was an established habit. "Wow," she said, "you're really serious about running, that's great." I walked away feeling the pleasant pricklings of pride until I realized she thought "ten" meant ten *miles*, not ten kilometers. I had never run ten miles in my life! I had misrepresented myself— unwittingly of course, but I was still mortified.

I went home, put on my shorts and shoes, and went to the park. I did one loop. Ten kilometers. Or as I was now trying to think of it, six miles. I did a second loop. Twenty kilometers. That was twelve miles. Wow. My conversion math was getting better.

My feet hurt. My hips felt misaligned. Salt caked my temples. My skin tingled and my hair stood on end. My lungs expanded and opened up, so that I breathed in an entire world at my disposal. I had just run the farthest I ever had in my life, twice over, and I felt amazing. Only a few hours earlier I wouldn't even have thought it was possible. It was as if I had opened a door to an alternate universe, my own Narnia, or Alice down the rabbit hole. What next? I thought, newly plugged into a high voltage of potential. What do I think I *can't* do? I'll do that! Maybe, I thought, there was no such thing as an I-can-only-dream-of list.

I was addicted.

"What next? I thought, newly plugged into a high voltage of potential. What do I think I *can't* do?"

Sure, the more-than-good feeling after that first twelve-mile run could have been the endorphins, but I think it was more.

Rain, snow, or shine; dark mornings and sunny afternoons; exploring a new city or a forest path; ever since that day, running has given me freedom and strength. The energy it generates courses through the arteries of my life, oxygenating my dreams.

I started the run with no more than an idea of reclaiming my secretly eroded integrity. After all, the likelihood that my hoped-for-friend would ever learn I ran less than she'd thought was close to nil. Yet somehow I could not let my misrepresentation lie. In the process I proved to myself that I had *no idea* what I was capable of. I saw with new clarity how much I had underestimated my own ability.

Marathon?—I can do that!

So I did.

I ran another and another.

And along the way I started to make changes in the rest of my life. If I could do the seemingly impossible—run a marathon—what else could I do?

There is something profoundly liberating about this quintessential running achievement. It's as if in accomplishing it, we not only surpass a performance threshold that now redefines us as an athlete, but we also have exceeded our own threshold of personal limitation. A marathon, and most other benchmark athletic accomplishments, become watershed moments for many of us, perhaps because our bodies take us to a place our minds thought they couldn't go. And our mind, unconfined, throws open the door to enormous personal potential.

As Sally Friedman wrote in her book, *Swimming the Channel,* about the death of her husband and the dissolution of her plans to swim the English Channel, "When we have done something beyond the realm of normal middle-class life, something out of the ordinary, the unexpected, it becomes, '[A] secret source of confidence, a private wellspring of originality.'"

So many women I interviewed spoke of their marathon accomplishment in similar terms—"If I can do a marathon, I can do anything." Kathrine Switzer says she felt hugely empowered when she became the first woman to conquer the Boston Marathon, her first. As she still says, "If I'm facing something new or difficult, I just think to myself, if I can shake off Jock Semple [former Boston Marathon director] as he tries to pull me off the marathon course, I can do anything."

The same holds true for nonelite runners like the rest of us. Take Rebecca Yzquierdo, for example. Until she started training for her first marathon, Rebecca says she often identified herself as a helpless woman in emergency situations. Running changed, not only her view of herself as an athlete, but also her belief that she could rise to a challenge. Here's an example I like, especially because I've never yet had the gumption to do what Rebecca did when faced with a triple-A moment. On her way to the mall in her native Houston one day, Rebecca drove over a ladder in the middle of the freeway and barely made it into the parking lot with a flat tire. She went looking for a man to help her, but not even the security guard was willing to come to her rescue. She felt a panic attack

"'If I can run a marathon, I can totally change this tire.'"

coming, so she took a deep breath and said to herself, "If I can run a marathon, I can totally change this tire." Out came the car manual and lo and behold, she changed the tire. Her last thought: "I knew then I was capable of many things."

Our running shoes have magic in them—the power to transform a bad day into a good day; frustration into speed; self-doubt into confidence; chocolate cake into muscle; or, as in Rebecca's case, a flat tire problem into an accomplishment.

THIS IS YOUR BRAIN ON EXERCISE

We know from experience that our sports energize us and give us confidence—in ourselves and our ability to fully realize the vitality and possibility of our lives. And now science is catching up with what we know viscerally to be true.

In *Spark: The Revolutionary New Science of Exercise and the Brain*, Harvard psychology professor John Ratey shows how exercise actually builds and conditions our brains so that we learn better, are happier and healthier, and can age more gracefully. His goal is to show how the mind and body are not separate entities, they are connected.

We know this because we've literally felt that connection at times.

In his book, Ratey covers a range of topics, showing in each case how exercise improves cognitive abilities and mental health issues; in other words, how exercise improves learning and ameliorates conditions as diverse as depression, anxiety disorders, ADHD, menopause, Alzheimer's, Parkinson's, and yes, aging in general. Ratey shows how exercise literally helps the brain grow. How great is that? And here's a cool word to go with it: neurogenesis. Now we can say we're going out to "neurogenesize" instead of exercise. Which is especially reassuring considering that the human brain starts to lose nerve tissue beginning at age thirty.

As Ratey writes, "The neurons in the brain connect to one another through 'leaves' on treelike branches, and exercise causes those branches to grow and bloom with new buds, thus enhancing brain function at a fundamental level." And later he writes this of the spark that exercise ignites in us: "It lights a fire on every level of your brain, from stoking up the neurons' metabolic furnaces to forging the very structures that transmit information from one synapse to the next."

That deserves a moment's pause to consider the implications: exercise, it seems, is Miracle-Gro fertilizer for our brain. No more "dumb jock"—we're getting smarter with every workout.

 "[E]xercise, it seems, is Miracle-Gro fertilizer for our brain."

Ratey, of course, goes into much more detail about the biological and chemical effects of exercise. I need to run a bit more before my brain grows enough new "leaves" to retain all the acronyms (vascular endothelial growth factor [VEGF], for example).

When we pursue our sports, we not only feel happier, we're simultaneously tapping into and replenishing our reserves of strength, courage, flexibility, and stamina—not just physically, but mentally and emotionally. We certainly *feel* the connection and the benefits. Who hasn't experienced the classic "runner's high" (which can happen during any significant physical effort) and felt the moment our bodies released endorphins, those euphoria-inducing, pain-killing biochemicals that have properties similar to morphine? There's more.

Exercising at high intensity also increases epinephrine, which can be depleted by stress and anxiety, causing fatigue. So more exercise equals more epinephrine, which means more energy, juicing us back up after stressful days. Vigorous exercise does the same for levels of serotonin, a mood-lifting neurochemical associated with contentment that is also depleted when we are overly stressed, anxious, or undernourished. And note, research shows that low-carb dieters need to watch out for the latter. No wonder eating the whole breadbasket at a restaurant makes me so happy— it's a serotonin party for my body!

Research also shows that the rise in serotonin we experience from moderate-intensity workouts is comparable to the serotonin boost that comes from being surrounded by good friends and family we love. And finally, there's dopamine, the brain's "pleasure chemical," which is also released through exercise (and food, sex, and drugs). When triggered, it motivates us to pursue that activity more—in this case, more exercise—a healthier "addiction" all around. Thus, each time we run, we're conditioning ourselves physiologically to reward our brain with feelings of wellness and joy. Not to mention that our rewarded brains are neurogenesizing, too.

Suffice to say that the sports we pursue are good for us in more ways than we knew. Not that we need science to validate how we feel, but I find it grounding that science is catching up.

Mary Wittenberg, president and chief executive of New York Road Runners, puts it this way, "It's like a secret, that this activity [running] can transform your life in more ways than you know."

"'It's like a secret, that this activity [running] can transform your life in more ways than you know.'"

Not just running, but any sport pursued with purpose.

Mary's epiphany came during college when she was a cheerleader. Feeling sidelined and out of the game, literally, she took up rowing instead. When she wrote a letter to her father telling him about her decision to quit the squad, his response was incredulous: "Why would you do *that?*"

Despite her father's views, Mary traded her pom-poms for oars and discovered her own transformative secret. In the last twenty strokes of every rowing race, when she was at her limit and pulling harder still, that's when she realized how far she could really go. "The body," Mary says, "can go way farther than your mind thinks it can."

Mary is a great example of how the pleasure and benefits derived from exercise aren't just a result of our neurons exploding like a Fourth of July fireworks show, or even our brains growing like spring trees in leaf. There's another level of connection between the body and mind that athletes, dancers, martial artists, yoga enthusiasts, and others have practiced for ages that involves the *conscious* control of how we engage our muscles and bodies when we move.

It's called "somatic movement," and it, too, has an immense impact on how we feel, both physically and emotionally.

"Who we are is how we move," says Michelle Gay, a Certified Laban Movement Analyst and founder of the Society for Martial Arts Instruction. Her work as a sensei (a martial arts instructor) and movement teacher is to help others understand and tap into the very sources of how they move.

"Movement is 'somatic,'" says Michelle, who defines it as the deepest connection between our body and mind. It includes our reflexes, our instinctive movements (like fight or flight), the hardwiring of our system, as well as the developmental stages of movement.

"When we understand explicitly the nature of what *literally* moves us, then we discover choices we didn't know we had before." And by that she means, not only how we physically move, but also as it translates to the rest of our world.

In other words, when we move with intentional confidence, that physical approach to the world informs our emotional and psychological approach to the world. When we stand up straight, with our shoulders back, it widens our chests and opens our hearts. There's literally more room to breathe, and there's more room to expand into the world. To turn the familiar children's warning on its head, you *can* try this at home. The next time you are feeling low, consciously take a deep breath and straighten up, wherever you are, sitting or standing or lying down. Make new space for your heart and you will feel a new flow of positive energy.

Cool, right? I knew you'd feel the difference.

Who we are is how we move.

From running came the power to change myself, to move toward my dreams.

I quit the practice of law to become a writer. My hands shook as I made that life-altering call. My shirt was glued to my underarms with more sweat than an autumn run. I felt like I was launching into my future on an exploratory space probe—it might blow up, or it might discover a new planet. Because not only was I giving up a clear career trajectory and a handsome salary, stepping

"I felt like I was launching into my future on an exploratory space probe—it might blow up, or it might discover a new planet."

off the traditional path dictated by years of education, and entering a field in which I had no prior role models in my life—but I also faced a deeply entrenched psychological challenge: all through my undergraduate degree and into law school, I dreaded all writing assignments. The fact that I did well never assuaged my fears. I was convinced that I was a terrible writer. But I hadn't always thought that way. In fact, I was a writer long before I was runner.

EAT MY DUST, MR. E!

When I published my first novel in 2007, my father sent me a photograph he'd taken when I was six. I was seated yogi-style on our front steps, selling not lemonade but my so-called "volumes." I'd stapled these handwritten pages together to constitute books, and I was offering to sell them to my neighbors for a nickel apiece. They were titled *The Girl's Book*, *The Boy's Book*, and *The Girls and Boys Book*, and they detailed the kinds of things each gender liked to do. Building with LEGOs featured in all the books, as did playing outside. But while the girls got dresses to wear, the boys were relegated to diapers—having two younger brothers had its influences, and I was quite the expert diaper changer. By the age of twelve, I'd built up my writing endurance from staple-books to a full-fledged play, which I wrote for my Hebrew school class. As I recall, we even performed it as a kind of shadow Chanukah play behind a scrim.

At an age where a whole body of research shows that teens are developing clear ideas about potential career paths, I knew exactly what I wanted to do. I was a writer, with some actress thrown in for good measure. Fast-forward to twelfth grade. My high school English teacher offered to read and comment on anything we wanted to write outside of class. The work wouldn't be graded and it wasn't a requirement. We were doing it for fun. I spent hours writing a short story I was enormously proud of, and when I turned it in, I was convinced I was the next Margaret Atwood. A few days later my story reappeared in my class folder with the red ink of comments. My heart in my throat, I couldn't wait to read his remarks. *Hmmm. Not much red.* Written across the top in a quick script was the following comment: "I don't think it's worthwhile for you to continue with this exercise. Focus instead on the class work." The whole world went silent, save for the rush of blood to my head. Mr. E said I didn't have the talent, and who was I to argue with his assessment? I gave up writing and studied to be a lawyer instead.

I had buried the writer part of myself, and when it came time to excavate her, the painstaking process of rediscovery required every self-archaeology tool at my disposal—scraping off my neglect-encrusted love of words, piecing together the fragments of my fear-lessness, and oiling my rusty imagination. Why was recapturing this lost piece of me so hard?—because our bodies and minds do not always cooperate with each other. Sometimes, despite our athletic-induced confidence, the mind will trip us up on the road to happiness by littering our path with obstacles, like a discouraging teacher's words that we've internalized as insecurity.

"Sometimes, despite our athletic-induced confidence, the mind will trip us up on the road to happiness. . . ."

The less we believe in our worth, the less we'll achieve—even with the occasional runner's high. Just as we have to train our bodies to be strong, we have to train our minds to be strong. Doing both in concert creates a positive feedback loop that becomes a powerful antidote against the disease of delusional can't-do thinking.

Katy Earhart, owner of an online women's sporting goods business, has her own "discouraging teacher" story. When she was a teenager, the small high school she attended had a policy that everyone who wanted to play on a team sport would be allowed to, regardless of their skill level. Unfortunately, Katie's small size made it difficult for her to shine on the basketball and volleyball courts alongside the taller, more robust girls. The coaches had no choice but to include her, yet according to Katy, they found every reason to keep her on the bench. On one occasion, she says, her volleyball coach even called an emergency time-out because he'd forgotten to deploy his usual tactic of rotating Katy off the court before she reached the serving position. The diversion didn't work, but that's not even the discouraging part of the story!

Another one of her teachers, "Mrs. B," called Katy and her equally athletically-sidelined best friend into her office for a chat. According to Katy, Mrs. B suggested that "little Katy" and her best buddy "find some new friends" and stop hanging around the athletic girls, where they didn't fit in. Katy and her friend obliged. After all, Mrs. B was the authority on what constituted athletic, and so Katy believed that despite her desires, she wasn't cut out for athletics.

Fast-forward almost a decade later. Katy is preparing to run her first marathon, having overcome the negative influences that drove her off the courts. Her high school best friend sends her a T-shirt that reads: "Eat my dust, Mrs. B!" Katy wears it to bed the night before the race and wakes up inspired, ready to dominate those 26.2 miles, which she does handily. A year later and Katy, who feels strongly about the empowerment possibilities of sports for women, starts a company that sells cool stuff—from technical running shirts to inspiring jewelry for women runners. One of the very first customers she has is, of all people, Mrs. B's daughter. A kind note from Mrs. B follows soon after, with congratulations on Katy's venture.

For Katy, it was better than any apology. She got to kick that discouraging teacher out of her mind once and for all.

Or take freelance writer Heidi Swift. She didn't even have a discouraging teacher whispering in her ear. Her mind was working its *own* invented agenda of negativity. Heidi "knew" she could never ride 100 miles on a bicycle. She was certain she didn't have the stamina to go the distance, both physically and psychologically.

"'What you know and what you think you know are both subject to what you will allow yourself to believe,' she says, adding, 'and "never" can kiss my saddlebag!'"

When friends convinced her to sign up for a century ride in Vancouver, British Columbia, she discovered she was way off course in her thinking.

"What you know and what you think you know are both subject to what you will allow yourself to believe," she says, adding, "and 'never' can kiss my saddlebag!"

LOOKING UNDER THE HOOD

One of the many things sports have taught me is to enjoy being alone with myself, to look inward and reflect. It's probably why I like meditation and the occasional dharma talk. That's Buddhist lingo for a talk about why we exist and how we might live more consciously, and therefore more harmoniously, in the world. I'm not Buddhist, but I like thinking about these things.

I think of it as "looking under the hood." Too many of us spend a good portion of our lives thinking we have control over things we don't have control over (like whether our new lover will actually fall in love with us) and that we have no say in the things we *do* have control over (such as whether we are happy). But if we open up the hood—and I'm thinking of the cartoon head that pops open like a PEZ candy dispenser during the surreal opening sequence to Monty Python's Flying Circus, revealing a circus of thoughts—we see that we have control over what's going on in the engine of our mind.

One such dharma talk I attended was given by Kadam Morten, the resident teacher at the Chakrasambara Buddhist Meditation Center in New York City. He spoke about our habit of negative thinking, which is so much more powerful than our habit of

"We forget that happiness and suffering are states of mind."

positive thinking. He pointed out that most of us identify much more closely with what we believe is our "bad," or negative, nature rather than our "pure," or good nature, which according to Buddhist philosophy is the essence of every human being.

We forget that happiness and suffering are states of mind.

According to Buddhist thought, negative or delusional thinking happens when we become too attached to the outer world and ascribe the power to make us happy to a "thing" we perceive with our mind, like another person, a possession, or an ambition. Instead we need to practice the central Buddhist principle of "nonattachment," to go with the flow by not resisting what comes our way; to disconnect our happiness from external sources and look inward for our happiness instead.

How can we know the difference between attachment and nonattachment? Well, my guess is that all of us have experienced the difference firsthand in our pursuit of goals in sports. My first marathon is a case in point. I started out running too fast, a classic mistake. From the fast start, I then proved out the mathematical formula my running coach had warned me about. "For every minute you're ahead of your time at the 10k, you'll be ten minutes behind at the finish." Indeed. I flew past 10k three minutes ahead of schedule, only to struggle across the finish line half an hour after my goal. I was so devastated by my "failure" that I refused to take the finisher's medal when the volunteer tried to put it around my neck. I thought I wasn't worthy.

The wires in my brain must have been crossed. Instead of enjoying the good feeling any first-time marathoner ought to feel crossing the finish line, my mind used the accomplishment as an opportunity to reinforce a negative identity.

As Geshe Kelsang Gyatso says in *Transform Your Life: A Blissful Journey*, "Happiness and suffering are states of mind, and so their main causes cannot be found outside the mind. The real source of happiness is inner peace. If our mind is peaceful, we will be happy all the time, regardless of external conditions, but if it is disturbed or troubled in any way, we will never be happy, no matter how good our external conditions may be."

How, then, do we counter our negative thinking? We shift our self-identification. For example, I might say, "I'm a writer," instead of, "Mr. E was right. I suck at writing and should never even try." Or this, "I just finished my first marathon, I'm amazing," instead of, "What kind of loser goes out too fast at the start of a long race?"

In other words, if we say, "I am a strong athlete," there's a good chance that's what we'll be. Sports psychologists call this "exercise identity." In *Sport and Exercise Psychology: The Key Concepts*, Ellis Cashmore defines this as being "when an adherent integrates

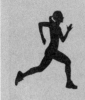

> "In other words, if we say, 'I am a strong athlete,' there's a good chance that's what we'll be."

the activity into his or her own conception of self. This affects practically every other aspect of a person's being."

When we identify ourselves as the kind of person who perseveres in the face of challenges on the road, we begin to see ourselves that way in life generally, too.

Kadam Morten pointed out that as we're making the transition to identifying with our good nature, it's important to be skillful about how we set our goals. A first-time runner who wants to finish their marathon in two and a half hours will likely be wildly disappointed, not to mention discouraged, and will reidentify with their "bad" nature. "I only ran a 3:45, what a wimp." To avoid setting ourselves up for failure, we must set realistic goals. Turn up the heat slowly. Think of putting all our negative identifications into a pot of cold water and slowly boiling them away. Don't worry. They won't notice until it's too late.

Carrie Barrett is a great example of proof in action. At twenty-four, the stand-up comic had just moved to Austin, Texas. With her heart recently broken and lonely in a new town, she was eating too much and drinking too much. At fifty pounds overweight, she felt blue about life, and life had barely begun. This was not the way she wanted to live out the rest of her twenties. She took stock of her life and realized that she desperately needed a physical and emotional change—a permanent one. So she set herself a goal:

to run a marathon by age thirty. Mustering her courage—which she had on tap from doing stand-up comedy—she signed up for a beginning running group. The catch: she had never run before. *Ever.* She worried she'd be the biggest, slowest person in the group (she was neither) or stand out and embarrass herself in some other way (no, again). In short, she didn't identify herself as a runner yet. She identified herself as an overweight, out-of-shape person, though one who was going to try her hand at running. Four years later— and two years shy of her goal—she crossed her first marathon finish line. At that moment, she says, the transformation was complete. She finally identified herself as an athlete. In the seven years since, she's done fifteen marathons, a slew of triathlons, and an Ironman. She also gives back to the sports she loves by volunteering at races, raising money for charities through racing, and coaching others to accomplish their own extraordinary athletic goals. She flicked the self-identification switch in her head to the positive setting, and it's been on ever since.

Carrie says she sometimes misses the "buzz" of her first few races, the thrill and surprise that would come from simply *finishing* each race.

I know what she means. I remember my first triathlon. I'm dating myself, but it was back in 1993. It was a short race, something that might take me little more than an hour now. I didn't know another person who did triathlons. They weren't that popular yet, certainly not with women. I had used swim goggles only three times in my life. (Who knew it took so much skill just to prevent them from leaking?) In the first moments of the mass-start swim, someone kicked them off my face. I straggled in from the swim and spent inordinate time collecting my wits and preparing to tackle the bike portion of the race. I pedaled hard into last place on my heavy mountain bike and ran slightly better to finish in second to last place.

For a few days I felt like a rock star. I purposely wore sleeveless tops so I could show off my new strong arms. Thankfully for my retrospective self-esteem, I stopped short of flexing my biceps in that guy-who-pumps-iron way. But the rock star feeling didn't last. The negative messages were still too loud. I wasn't really that woman who had finished that race. Instead, I thought of myself as just having "pretended" for the day. You know, "I'm not a doctor, I just play one on TV." But the triathlon was a precursor, a beacon maybe, of the twelve-mile run yet to come. I still didn't see myself as an athlete, and certainly not as a writer. But all that came in time.

 "For a few days I felt like a rock star. I purposely wore sleeveless tops so I could show off my new strong arms."

Flicking the switch isn't easy. Sure, it *sounds* simple. Be strong, physically, emotionally, and psychologically, and you will be happier. Send yourself the right positive messages and you'll have more energy and zeal for your whole life—to ask for that promotion or raise, to follow your passion instead of playing it safe, or start your own business—to really *live*. After all, why coast through life when you can run, skip, or jump? As Lois, the flight attendant in her early sixties, says, "I want to get on life's page."

So how do we do it? Well, one good place to start is through "visualizing."

WYSIWYG

I recently read that "Your imagination can be trained like a muscle." That is to say, the more we visualize our own bright future, the better we'll get at it. In *Thinking Body, Dancing Mind: Taosports for Extraordinary Performance in Athletics, Business, and Life*, coauthors Chungliang Al Huang and Jerry Lynch point out that "Acting 'as if' you can achieve something is self-direction, not self-deception." Good to know that visualizing isn't hallucinating. It's creating an intention with the deepest of roots.

Our intrepid tire-changer, Rebecca, says she used visualization when she was training for her first marathon. At times she would be so overcome by visualizing the moment of finishing the race that she would start crying. At other times she'd find herself hyperventilating. Everything felt so exaggerated and new to her. "My body was doing things that it had never done before, and I was not only making new discoveries with it, I was reinventing myself to become the person I truly was, and the person I felt I was inside."

Rebecca discovered a new person within herself, and along the way she also lost over sixty pounds, discovering a new person on the outside, too.

Visualizing is equally powerful in any sport. Climbers will "think" about a rock face before they climb. They'll imagine reaching for a hold and finding the small outcrop or crack or unevenness in the rock. I've had yoga instructors who suggest that before doing a pose, we first imagine *being* in that pose, "feeling" the balance and alignment in our body before actually doing the pose. I once knew a woman who spent an entire summer watching downhill ski videos and visualizing herself swishing down the slope. When the snow fell that winter, her skiing had improved dramatically.

Sports is not the only place where we can visualize positive outcomes. Visualizing can apply to anything difficult, challenging, or hard to reach. If we can "see" and own our hopes, dreams, and ambitions, then we are far more likely to achieve them. In fact, some might say that believing in our dreams, which means we've "seen" them come true before they do, is the only way dreams come true. "What you see is what you get," or "WYSIWYG," as the computer-world acronym goes, an expression used to describe programs and applications that work in obvious, intuitive ways.

Visualizing is a critical source of confidence in the future.

 "If we can 'see' and own our hopes, dreams, and ambitions, then we are far more likely to achieve them."

When Holly Brooks, the twenty-seven-year-old cross-country skiing coach for Alaska Pacific University, first dared to think about the 2010 Winter Olympics, she was scared to say aloud what she was thinking. But in September 2009 she put her dream in writing, in an article for athleta.net titled, "I want to be an Olympian." She had said the "O" word in public. And what do you know? When Holly owned her goals, when she "saw" or "visualized" her future, she achieved her dream, winning a much-coveted place on the Olympic team.

In *Body Mind Mastery: Training for Sport and Life*, author Dan Millman puts it this way, "Visualize your dreams in detail. Your subconscious mind doesn't clearly differentiate between what you visualize in your mind's eye and what you see with your physical eye, so the more you visualize positive outcomes, the more you attract them into your life."

I was relieved to read about visualizing in detail. Otherwise I might have called some of my visualization straight-up fantasizing instead. As in, I'm daydreaming about promoting my book on television . . . *Should I wear flats? Do I own any nice ones? Or heels—more flattering, but must be weighed against the trip-and-fall danger . . .*

As much as we need to visualize our dreams, we know from Buddha that we shouldn't get too attached to them. And he had a pretty good handle on what's what. If I'm never on television, that's perfectly fine. Because if our dreams don't quite turn out the way we thought, well then, we could be back to the same old cycle of negative messages. To wit, recall my excessive attachment to my first marathon goal, which prevented me from enjoying my accomplishment. Instead, visualize and let go.

As Lynn, a forty-eight-year-old devotee of all mountain sports points out, that process is exactly like climbing. "When you start at the bottom of a climbing route, you can't see all the holds you're going to use, you can't see the exact route you're going to follow, and half the time you can't see where the top is either. You move up one little step at a time . . . I've learned a lot about being me, and about *who* me is, in the mountains. When I climb a peak that scares me, I feel afterward that I could accomplish anything."

 "'When I climb a peak that scares me, I feel afterward that I could accomplish anything.'"

Within each of us exists the possibility of the extraordinary, to "be somebody." As Lily Tomlin once said, "I always wanted to be somebody, but maybe I should have been more specific." Lily T did just fine without the specifics. For the rest of us, we need to work hard to find and keep our own extraordinary possibility current in our lives.

IT'S YOUR LIFE, DON'T MISS IT!

Once we know our minds are what limit our capacity, and not our capacity setting the limits, then we've opened up a world of possibility.

Reimagining ourselves as someone new—an athlete, say—has wildly invigorating potential.

Kathrine Switzer told me about seeing the "I am somebody" realization click on a first-time marathoner's face when the finisher's medal was put around her neck. At women's running clinics around the United States, she's encountered women who are sullen, embarrassed by their weight, or barely willing to participate (they've been dragged there in the first place by someone else).

"I tell them they're not too old, too fat, too slow, too ignorant, whatever it is they are telling themselves," says Kathrine.

Crossing the finish line changes everything. They finally believe in themselves. In Brazil, for example, Kathrine's seen how it can transform the very culture and society. Women come out in startling numbers for all-women's races, and once they've crossed the finish line they are unstoppable. They start their own businesses. They find their own lives.

They become writers.

Wait—that's *me*.

Reimagining myself as an athlete helped me to reimagine myself as a writer instead of a lawyer, to shrug off not only my suits but also the yoke of more than a few fixed beliefs.

I started writing—or should I say writing *again*—almost by accident. In a pause between careers, right after I'd made the decision to stay in New York and leave the practice of law, I took a writing class on a whim. I like learning new things. Being a beginner has its frustrations, but it also has its rewards. Developing new skills always brings a certain thrill with it. Over the years, I've taken cooking, photography, ballet, hip hop, guitar, painting, singing, and pole dancing, just to name a few.

I signed up for a beginner class called "How to Write a Short Story" at my neighborhood YMCA. I had no expectations beyond a brief diversion while I was job hunting. I was so wrong. My renewed relationship with writing was love at first ink.

In the very first class we began "training" with free-writing exercises. This is on-the-spot writing, either completely free form or on a specific topic, generally done for a certain length of time or number of pages. I looked at my blank, ruled page that first evening in class and my mind emptied. What to write? Had I ever had a thought in my life? All my life my brain had felt cluttered—chatter, chatter, chattering at me—and suddenly my mind was quiet. But I wasn't worried. For the first time in a while, I had no agenda. If I was no good at this writing thing, there was nothing lost. Then, like the first vapors of steam from a kettle set to boil, images gathered force, until I was compelled to write them down. A story formed of a deaf girl who played the cello. I had never known anyone deaf, nor had I known any cello players.

I had discovered my imagination. And like the strength we discover in sports, once you've caught a glimpse of your own hidden resources, there's no hiding from them. The cat won't be put back in the bag. And who would want to put the cat away anyway? Or their strength for that matter, *or* their imagination?

 "[T]o be strong in body and mind requires not only effort but also risk and the willingness to embrace a new mind-set."

As I became a stronger runner—not to mention, cyclist, swimmer, climber, skier, kayaker, and more—I also became surer of my writing. Believing in myself isn't always easy, but it is the effort—the training and the writing—that bring me the most sustained happiness. That is the joy.

Yet to be strong in body and mind requires not only effort but also risk and the willingness to embrace a new mind-set.

Was it scary to make the leap, to leave the practice of law and pursue an entirely new career? Absolutely terrifying but exciting and liberating as well. Risk has a way of making the heart beat faster, much like in sports. In both cases, accelerating the heart rate can have salutary effects, physically and emotionally. We find what we think is our limit and we push, and then we push again, giving us the power to change our lives in profound ways.

Meg Benson knows this intimately.

After having two children, Meg's childhood scoliosis flared up so badly that x-rays of her spine showed what looked like a

"She felt cornered, without any escape route. And that's just when things started to get better."

colony of mushrooms instead of a column of healthy vertebrae. She was plagued by constant and excruciating pain and could hardly walk. The extensive medical care she required was prohibitively expensive, and she didn't qualify for disability. The doctors told her she was destined to be in a wheelchair. Meanwhile, she had two young daughters to raise, a small jewelry shop to run in her hometown in Vermont, and a half-finished, uninhabitable house that she and her husband were building by hand. They were living in the garage as a temporary solution.

She felt cornered, without any escape route. And that's just when things started to get better.

"Being turned down for disability was the best thing that ever happened to me," Meg says now. "It closed off all the options except one—me. If there was a solution to my problems, it was me. No one else was going to fix me. I was responsible for my own health."

Instead of giving up or giving in, Meg fought. Lying on the floor one day she was determined to exercise her back and regain her strength. She pushed into the pain, relentlessly exercising when others weren't around to witness her contortions. One day she decided to try riding her bicycle again. She crawled out of her house, dragging her bike with her. Alone on a quiet country road, she laid her bike down on the ground and lifted a leg over to straddle it. Slowly she righted the bicycle beneath her and began to coast down the hill.

She couldn't pedal. It was too painful. As she reached the first inter-section, still unable to pedal, she had a choice. Turn right and keep coasting downhill until pedaling might be possible, or stop and fall sideways off the bike and then somehow make her way home.

She kept going.

After two miles of coasting, she found her ability to pedal. Her cycling form wasn't pretty and it didn't feel good. The ride was grueling, disheartening, humiliating, and frustrating. She spent the next year on her home-invented exercises to strengthen her back and what passed for riding her bike in that period. The road to re-covery took more than a year, paved with sheer will. But it worked.

When you walk into Meg's shop now, filled with the gorgeous jewelry she has designed and created, you'll find a beautiful, strong, straight-backed woman full of energy and a zeal for life, biking in the summer, telemark skiing in the winter. Has she looked at an x-ray of her back lately? She doesn't need to, she feels great.

Strength, energy, zeal, passion, vitality—just saying the words can feel daunting and, yes, risky. We need courage to make them a way of living. Like Meg, so many of the women's stories I heard had some element of fearlessness to them.

To be fearless, now that's a trick—facing risk with cour-age. We are born fearless and then little by little the boldness gets squeezed out of us, that is, until we learn to run like a girl and reclaim our natural life force.

Keri Fullmer, a project director and statistician at the Na-tional Institute of Health, was deathly afraid of water. She never put her head under the running water in the shower, and if she entered water up to her chest she would hyperventilate. No surprise that she didn't learn how to swim until she was thirty-five. The surprise is that she learned to swim at all. Like so many of her friends, she wanted to do a triathlon. The catch: to do the race she had no choice but to learn to swim. And she was done feeling embarrassed that she couldn't do something that seemed so effortless for others.

"I literally had to learn how to blow bubbles in kids' toys," says Keri of her first swimming lesson. "A little humiliating, but well worth it." Now Keri's done her first triathlon, and more are in the offing.

There's no add-water-and-stir instant recipe for running like a girl. For me, embracing my RLAG spirit took years, and it keeps on growing. Along the way there have been different peaks, moments when I believed that *little* bit more in myself. One peak that stands out is my eighth marathon.

I trained hard and I felt strong. But I'd seen that movie before—the one where I'd done everything right but didn't get the race right. As a friend of mine says, this was not my first rodeo.

So I needed an extra amount of courage to believe in my ability to do the best marathon I was capable of. At first I didn't even want to state my goal out loud. For starters, it was preposterous, much faster than I'd ever run a marathon before. Then one day running with my longtime training partner and close friend, Tammy, I was able to say the words aloud:

"I want to run a 3:16."

It practically scared the running shorts right off me to say the words aloud, to "own" the ambition. I second-guessed myself almost immediately. Wondering if I'd made a mistake by letting anyone in the world know what I thought I was capable of. But owning my ambition felt right. I knew in my heart I could make that time, even if race day didn't work out as I planned. And what do you know? I

"It practically scared the running shorts right off me to say the words aloud, to 'own' the ambition."

actually beat my own scary goal. At the age of forty-two, after seven previous marathons, I surpassed all my personal bests by a whopping 15 minutes and did a 3:14 marathon, coming in twentieth out of the nearly one thousand women who ran the race.

When I started that race I could feel the possibility of its outcome in my whole body. Literally. When the starting gun sounded, my nerve endings tingled on the surface of my skin, the muscles in my legs twitched in anticipation. I felt a wave of almost-tears wash through me.

I whispered to myself, "You can do it. Go for it."

I'm so tired. Have I been this tired before? That eighth marathon is a distant memory and sometimes I wonder how I ever did it. My legs don't hurt. It's more like they've been zap-gunned by space invaders into slow motion. I tap my watch and recalculate. It really *did* take me five minutes longer to run this ascent than last week. I feel as if time just disappeared, and where was I? Did I take a catnap on the trail without noticing? That almost seems possible.

Pikes Peak. The difficulty of the "I-could-never-do-that" race I'm training for is beginning to overwhelm me. Running thirteen miles up nearly eight thousand feet of mountain trails? And that's only the first half. Then there's the down. As I struggle to maintain my pace, I wonder when the universe shifted and I went from saying, "no way" to "when's the sign-up day?" And this is it. My last long training run before the event, and I'm profoundly exhausted. . . .

As I reach the summit, a wave of terror washes through me out of nowhere, like the flush of a near car crash, followed by every nerve ending in my body a-fizz with the tremors of that near miss. *I can't do this race!* My whole body feels weightless for a second, and then statue-stone heavy. My feet shuffle. My body twists. I wrench myself upright from an almost-trip over one of the treacherously loose rocks on the path. I stop and turn 360 degrees, slowly, gulping in the green hills with their filigree of trails, the gray peaks squatted in the blue sky.

The downhill goes more slowly than usual, too. Running through the shin-high mule's ears a mile or so from the end, my body feels hollowed out with hunger and I half expect to hear my organs rattling around inside me.

At the car I fumble with the clip on my camelback, then sink into the driver's seat. When I turn on the radio, Green Day's song, "Boulevard of Broken Dreams," comes on the radio and my eyes well up with tears, *Will my shadow run beside me?* I know other people do these races and harder. But I'm not them. Or they're not me. *I can't do this race.*

I breathe. I remind myself of the poet Rumi's words, "If all you can do is crawl, start crawling."

Because here is what I know for certain—I can't finish the race if I don't start. And that answers the question.

I *can* do this. I *am* possibility.

I'm going to start.

CHAPTER 3:

Rising to the (Almost) Daily Challenge

"Today is your day. Your mountain is waiting, so get on your way!"
—Dr. Seuss, author and illustrator

The sky is still dark, even though your alarm went off. It's cold outside and warm in bed. Maybe your husband, your child, your cat, or your fabulous new lover is curled up against you. Perhaps you stayed out too late last night, and you had that one more glass of wine. Or you couldn't stop reading the new Stieg Larsson mystery. Or you're worn out from work, from seeing friends, from kids, from life stress.

Today may be the first day of the rest of your life, but it also might be the 183rd day of your current workout regimen. Every fiber of your being groans, "Do I *have* to get up? Couldn't I skip the workout just this morning?"

Like eating and sleeping, or fostering friendships and a career, our athletic pursuits demand ongoing, often daily, attention. Sure, we may finish the event we've been training for all spring, but that doesn't mean we hang up our shoes once we cross the finish line. Maybe we reduce the intensity, take a break, or switch to a different sport. Ultimately, we come back to our sport because we reap enormous benefits from rising to the daily challenge of sticking to our workout plan. And lest you are thinking to yourself, "Daily?—I think not!" I don't mean daily *literally*. Daily is simply the word that captures the essence of our commitment, whether it's Monday, Wednesday, and Saturdays, or every day except Tuesday. Daily is each of us rising to the level we've set for ourselves.

Why rise?

Because the process of nourishing ourselves physically feeds into the rest of our lives, nourishing us mentally and emotionally in a cycle of increasing physical strength, psychological resilience, and hardihood of spirit.

As Katrine Strickland, a triathlete who works in advertising, says, "My morning workout is the hardest part of my day. Whatever comes up next I can handle."

Meeting ourselves daily on the road, in the pool, on the court, or in the bike saddle requires ongoing discipline.

Discipline?! I know. Even the word can sound exhausting. And that daily meet-up with sports can be especially hard because the rewards may seem less immediate and concrete than, say, the payroll deposit into your account. Yet, we do it to be healthier, happier, and more fulfilled; great reasons, just a little less tangible when the alarm goes off. To stick with it, we each need to find our own way to commit to the discipline.

One of the most direct and obvious ways in which we can do this is by setting goals for ourselves. Whether our aim is to do our first 5k trail run or to best our marathon time, these future goals anchor us to the dailyness of achieving them. Yet even as we set goals, we need to learn to deal with the inevitable disappointments, the obstacles to achieving them—both in and out of our control; or worse, the burnout that threatens if we focus too much on a Goal, and lose sight of the sheer pleasure of the training. Because remember, why do we participate? Don't tell me you've forgotten already. We do it for *fun,* because it makes us happy. When we run like a girl, we feel empowered. We feel strong. We are happy. We see a bigger world of opportunity. We do it for the sheer, unadulterated joy of propelling ourselves through time and space with the amazing gift the universe has given us: our bodies.

So why is it so ridiculously hard sometimes to keep at our sports? Why is the daily challenge just that, a challenge—almost every day?

GETTING OUR FRICTION ON

Sticking to this "hardest part of our day" on a regular basis operates something like the principle of inertia, which the did-an-apple-just-fall-on-my-head physicist Isaac Newton captured in his first law of motion several hundred years back. That is, an object in motion (in this case, us doing our workout, or perhaps not) will continue moving at its present speed or velocity. Great, except . . . if we're not moving—presto!—we're still not moving. Where our present speed equals zero, the principle of inertia says our future speed will also be zero; hence the difficulty of getting out of bed.

Present speed = Sleeping

Therefore:

Future speed = Sleeping

Inertia is only interrupted by *friction*, a change in the stability of the environment (like our alarm clock) changing our condition from sleeping to waking, at which point we think to ourselves, "Time to get up and . . ." And what? Well, and *work out*. And then the principle of inertia takes over again in a lovely example of cause and effect. If I've propelled myself into my workout, I'm already moving, moving, moving as I get into the rest of my day. We don't think of inertia as including motion, but it does. That's why it feels easier to continue a workout once we've started.

That's also why if you prefer your workouts at the end of the day, then you probably find it easier to exercise right when you get home, or maybe even before you go home. How much harder is it to get off the comfy couch once you've plopped down on it after work? If *I* do that, it's usually a case of "FLW" or "famous last words." As in, "Just give me a couple of minutes on the couch and then I'll work out."

Rest assured, on most occasions it would be a safe bet that you'd still find me on the couch an hour later. Unless I can find a source of friction—a running date with a friend, for example; or more pressing still, the need to pick up my child.

Cindy Parker is a serious runner with serious time constraints, which got even tighter after her daughter was born. Her solution? Every day, she'd take her daughter the five miles to her daycare center using the baby jogger. From there she'd head to work and then pick her back up for the five-mile run home. In case you're counting, that's a fifty-mile week, and that's *before* the weekend has even arrived. Cindy's friction was the necessity of transportation—her daughter had to get to daycare, and they both had to get home at the end of the day.

Like Cindy, our discipline is our friction, coaxing us to get moving, day in and day out. Once we've developed our routine, we know how valuable that regularity can be.

Jodi Bailey's sport is mushing (dog sled racing). She trains six to twelve hours a day, often in the dark, since she's training in Alaska. Boredom, sleep deprivation, and far too much time alone with nobody's voice but her own (if only her dogs could talk),

"A body not in motion, well, doesn't go anywhere."

means she needs to stay positive, not to mention sane. But Jodi has the added commitment, or incentive—depending on how you look at it—of having a kennel of forty to fifty sled dogs to raise and train for the grueling, several-hundred-mile-long, sub-zero-temperature races she does with them. In Jodi's case, the dogs are her friction, spurring her along. At the same time, she says, "I don't take myself too seriously." And it doesn't hurt to have a get-out-there attitude. As she says, "If it can be done, I can do it."

Life's a challenge. How nice if we could get through it with strength and grace. Or we could do nothing that challenges us, ever. A body not in motion, well, doesn't go anywhere. It simply rusts in place, like the Tin Man in *The Wizard of Oz*.

Why?—because our bodies are granted to us on a "use it or lose it" basis, as Michelle Theall, former editor-in-chief of *Women's Adventure Magazine*, says. And sports are only one example of this principle, which applies to just about every facet of life. The more we use our minds, the sharper they are. The kinder we are to people, the more kindness is ingrained in our way of being. What happens when we stop using the French we learned in high school? You see my point—time for a manicure so the fingernails look good when we're pointing to things on the menu in Paris, hoping the food is something palatable.

Michelle has an intimate knowledge of the importance of fighting static inertia. She didn't have what you might call an encouraged beginning in sports. When at age ten she discovered her lifelong passion for running, her mother told her that if she played sports her ovaries might fall out. Wow. But she persisted anyway. Then when she was barely past thirty, Michelle was diagnosed with multiple sclerosis (MS). So she knows what she's talking about when she says, "Sports are a good base for anything that might hit you from left field."

Michelle doesn't know how her MS might have affected her if she hadn't had sports in her life. What she does know is that she needs to keep asking her body to go the distance. MS, as she explains, is all about signals that aren't getting through. But Michelle has learned that if she keeps sending the signals over and over again, then eventually the signals reach their destination in her body. As Michelle points out, "I'm just working with an extreme version of what most of us face in the process of aging. As we get older, for example, we lose agility. Why? Because we're older, yes, but much more important, because we no longer play the games we did as children, which required us to use our agility."

Use it or lose it. Michelle brings whole new meaning to "rising to the daily challenge."

"I can't say what sports means to me," she says now. "It *is* me."

Who we are is how we move. Michelle personifies the concept of "exercise identity," demonstrating how our physical strength is integrated into our very being and then we identify with our own power.

The very dailyness of the commitment to our sports is one of the important things that help us believe in ourselves. Day in and day out, we are reminded that we had the fortitude to get out there, the strength to keep going. To live fully, in spite of life's landmines.

"For some, that daily reminder—that friction in action—can have unexpected consequences."

In the yogic tradition, the energy and austerity of this sort of discipline is captured by the term "tapas," not to be confused with the scrumptious small plates of food served at Spanish restaurants. A Sanskrit word, tapas translates as "the purifying heat." According to Gary Kraftsow in his book *Yoga for Transformation*, tapas is about "purifying and strengthening our systems through disciplines designed to reduce physical, emotional, and mental impurities." Tapas is the energy we bring to cutting through the distractions in our life, often manifested in our myriad conditioned responses and habitual actions, so we can bring our full attention to the present moment. The idea of tapas captures the mental and physical elements of our daily challenge. Dedicating to our sports is so much more than a physical commitment; it is deeply mental and emotional as well. It requires the energy of our bodies *and* of our minds.

For some, that daily reminder—that friction in action—can have unexpected consequences.

Jo Beckham, a lawyer in the New York district attorney's office, has been running since she was twenty-two years old. She's sixty-three now, so that's a very early start in the timeline of women's running. Women were not even allowed to run in the New York City Marathon when Jo first laced up her shoes. To say she loves running would be an understatement. Nine of those New York marathons later and she still cries every time she crosses the finish line. Running ranks as the top three most important things in her life, just after family and career.

Best of all, running may have literally saved her life.

In the late '70s, when Central Park was less of the jewel it is today, Jo was threatened by a man brandishing a knife as she was running to work. She was so incensed at having her daily run interrupted (not to mention that she didn't want to be late for work) that she turned on the man and yelled, "You better leave me alone!"

He did.

I can't guarantee that running will give you the power to ward off attackers like Jo did, but being athletic won't hurt.

Donna Green had a similar experience. About three years after she started practicing karate, she was walking to her ceramics studio, head in the clouds, when a man slammed into her and tried to steal her bag. Another woman might have been terrified into submission. Not Donna, who is a black belt in full-contact karate. Her training had rooted itself too firmly into her fibers. She turned automatically to her 45-degree posture, a pre-fighting stance, her upper body straight and strong, torso turned at a 45-degree angle to her attacker, her legs comfortably apart and loosely bent. She felt her feet connected to the ground. She felt the alignment and heft of her whole body as she dropped her weight into the earth. Her arms hung loose and easy at her sides. She lifted her gaze and looked her attacker in the eyes.

He turned tail and fled.

Just as animals do, Donna had grounded herself and sent a message. Without raising so much as a fist, she had let her attacker know that if he was going to engage her, it was going to take a lot more energy than he'd thought the moment before. She hadn't done any karate, at least not what we think of as martial arts—*wham, bam, zow, pow!* Donna had projected her *inner* strength, the composure that develops over the years of getting her friction on daily, of being in touch with her tapas, of being in touch with her *potential force.*

Every day, we need to nourish our inner—and outer—force.

Yet, simply embracing the knowledge that we'll "lose it" if we don't "use it" may not always be enough to motivate us into action. From time to time, most of us need other incentives to get out there. That's where having goals are important—whether they are personal ones, like logging a specific number of miles each week; or more public goals, like competing in a triathlon, finishing a century ride, or scoring during a soccer game.

BE YOUR OWN ORACLE

To have the life we want, we need to know what we want. Sounds simple, but it's amazing how often the future seems like something we divine from a crystal ball instead of something we create for ourselves. We are each our own Oracle at Delphi.

The specificity of the goals in sports is good practice for setting bigger life goals. As Heidi, the social worker and marathon runner, says, "Sports demonstrate the value of knowing what you want and therefore getting it." She adds further, "Achieving in sports helps you believe that you are deserving of a good life."

Double bonus.

In his seminal interview series *The Power of Myth* with Bill Moyers, the great American thinker Joseph Campbell said, "A vital person vitalizes. If you find where your own life is, then you will bring life to the world."

And how do we find where our life is? As Heidi pointed out, by knowing what we want and going for it. By setting goals and reaching for them. Or as Campbell says, through "trials and revelations." In daily-life speak that means setting and meeting challenges in our lives through which we test and expand the limits of our own capacity. One of the great self-testing grounds is sports. Sure, how we do in a marathon does not ultimately matter in the grand scheme of life. What *does* matter is how you approach the challenge and whether you do it at all. *And* how you discipline yourself to forge ahead when the going is rough, exhausting, or just plain tedious. The trial is the act of taking the risk that you might not achieve what you set out to do. Out of the risks come the revelations. All of these so-called "trials" that we come to know so intimately from sports—that I came to know after my watershed twelve-mile run in Central Park—help us to know ourselves, to find our life, and, by extension, to bring life to the world.

And that's the second part of Campbell's philosophy on trials and revelations. Energy is infectious—whether good or bad.

> "Others sense our vitality, and in a happy act of psychological osmosis, they feel vitalized in return."

When we tap in to the good energy of our lives, through setting and meeting challenges in our life and reaping the physical and spiritual benefits, we naturally spread that good energy around. Others sense our vitality, and in a happy act of psychological osmosis, they feel vitalized in return. In the process, you never know, you may inspire others to set their own goals. Energy is contagious: when we are vital, we vitalize others.

You've probably divined it already, but goals are really just an extension of visualization. They are the specific outcomes we visualize for ourselves, our inner oracle in action.

Sue Holloway, an Olympic kayaker and silver and bronze medalist in the 1984 games, says she rehearsed her race starts in her mind. If she made a mistake (in her mental race), she would go back and "see" it again and again until she "raced" it perfectly. She was visualizing exactly how she was going to achieve her Olympic goal.

We're not all going to be Olympians, but if we don't own what we want we're not going anywhere else, either. Visualizing our future through the goals we set for ourselves is one effective form of ownership.

I felt the power of this when I trained for my first marathon. My coach had us run the final mile of the marathon course repeatedly, imagining that we were finishing the race; in other words, *owning* the marathon goal.

I also once did a half-marathon where I visualized the clock at the first mile marker showing the pace I wanted to run. My partner, ever thoughtful, put a Post-it note on the hotel bathroom mirror the night before with my split time written on it and a big exclamation mark. When I actually passed the clock at the first mile and saw the exact time I'd wanted to do, to the second, I felt the hairs go up on the back of my neck. For the next six miles of that race, I hit the clock at the moment I'd visualized. Things ultimately fell apart in both races, but that's okay. I'd seen my goal, and the attempt was exhilarating.

Marta Gregory, a lawyer and former college ski racer turned marathoner, feels less intimidated and more resilient as a result of the sports she's done through her life. Although Marta stopped racing years ago, when she faces big moments in her legal career, she visualizes the pre-race nervousness she felt and remembers how well she performed in spite of it. In other words, she's visualizing an outcome.

"The nervousness prior to a track meet or a ski race is just like the nervousness of dealing with something like the LSAT or an important meeting at work," she says. Marta knows that having goals requires fortitude. "There's no opportunity to take the easy way out in ski racing," she points out. "There's a lot of sucking it up, whatever the weather, whatever else is going on in your life."

The good news is that when we hit an obstacle in training, it usually feels surmountable, less "important," than the obstacles we face in the rest of our life. Yet the more accustomed we become to facing and solving challenges in our training, the better able we are at surmounting the obstacles elsewhere in our lives.

As suffragist Susan B. Anthony once said, "I began to feel that myself plus the bicycle was precisely what had gained me a measure of success in life—it was the hardihood of spirit that led me to begin, the persistence of will that held me to my task, and the patience that was willing to begin again when the last stroke had failed."

Susan B. knew a thing or two about overcoming hurdles.

Setting goals, however, does not mean our future is foretold. They are simply a heading, a directional intent toward an end result. *How* we visualize our outcomes is what keeps us on course or derails us from our heading. Achieving our goal requires us to be present, and even more important, it requires us to believe in ourselves *and* a positive outcome.

For example, you train for a race. Hard. You follow your coach's instructions to the letter. You listen to your body. You eat healthy and get lots of sleep. Or maybe you don't, yet despite whatever is happening in your training, whether you're on target or off, you maintain a positive attitude about your race goal. That's right. You don't go into a race anticipating the worst. You don't start out by qualifying your performance. "If I even finish . . ." No. You say, "I'm going to finish in this time," or "I'm going to finish strong," or even just "I'm going to finish." No-brainer? Maybe. But it's amazing how even a little discouragement, like fretting over the residue of a lingering injury (aren't they all?!) or even a tanked workout can unbridle your negativity. If you spend all your energy anticipating the worst, you'll trash-talk your race right into the garbage can.

As a triathlete and coach, Kelly Williamson often reminds herself that 90 percent of any race comes down to what's between her ears. Of course, the training is critical, and she writes out her own and her athletes' training plans in several-week increments. But she knows that if they stick to only 80 percent of the plan, that's okay, because preparation will only get you so far if your mind can't take you the rest of the way.

I think of the negativity in my head (and yes, I have more than my share) in terms of Anne Lamott's static-filled radio station, K-Fucked, with which we're already familiar. One inner DJ tells us we're fabulous, we're talented, we can reach that goal, so why not get out of bed and go on a run. We *will* finish the race strong. And then there's that *other* voice, the shock-jock who tells us we're just not good enough, we suck, why bother. You might as well just hit the sleep button again. The negative voice, often the loudest of the two (in my head anyway), tries to keep us from experiencing the pleasure of the moment and sabotages our ambition and self-confidence in the bargain, which as Kelly pointed out, is as critical to our performance as our physical conditioning. Many of us tune into Radio KFKD at least sometimes. Since it's inevitable that we'll tune in, it's essential that we up the volume on the good voice and dial down the bad voice.

So then . . . what if we *don't* hit our goal time or we *don't* finish strong or even finish at all? Does the world end? Do we feel worse because we dared to set a goal we didn't meet instead of having no goal at all? Do people think less of us? Well, according to Radio KFKD the missed goal time is a catastrophe, our lives are probably over, and we should throw in the towel. Or we could cruise the radio waves to National Public Me Radio, where the rea-

 "Life is not an express train to success. Failures are inevitable station stops along our journey."

sonable announcer will tell you the *truth;* that no, the race doesn't define who we are forever. It barely defines us for the day. Life is not an express train to success. Failures are inevitable station stops along our journey.

By understanding that we are not the outcome, we can embrace it as a teacher. From each setback we learn something valuable. We become wiser, stronger, and more capable of development. That's Campbell's trials and revelations.

In researching for this book, I spoke with several women who were Olympic hopefuls at one time or another. In some cases, when *the* day came for their qualifying race, the stars did not align for them. The Olympics were snatched from their grasp. In others, the Olympics were a more distant goal, but a realistic dream all the same. These women's lives zoomed off on different trajectories. Who knows what their lives would have been like if they'd made the Olympic team. Better? Not necessarily. Just different.

When the Olympics eluded Mary Wittenberg due to an injury, for example, she became a lawyer, but then found her way back to running, heading up one of the biggest running clubs in the United States, the New York Road Runners. Of course, the Olympics were important to Mary, but she was not so attached to the goal that she couldn't see all the other possibility life had to offer. She loves her work and she loves her life, and isn't that as good as it gets?

There are so many ways we can be happy. A race is a day. It's our outlook that defines the quality of our life.

We have so much more control over the psychological setbacks we encounter than we think we do. Owning our ambitions and our future also means owning the power we have over our attitude and emotions.

And as it turns out, our mind may be an easier obstacle to conquer than the myriad external ones that can get in the way of us rising to the daily challenge.

WHEN IT RAINS *AND* POURS

What if we love our alarm? The dulcimer sound wakes us to a day we're eager to start. *Bring on my running shoes. I've got miles to go!* What if we've set goals and achieved them? What if we're perennially tuned in to KGrrrT instead of KFKD and we have a tiger in our tank? You *go* girl. And we fling open the door to . . . gale-force winds, sheets of rain, hailstones the size of figs. *Am I on the movie set of 2012?*

Some things are just not in our control. Everything from weather and injury to nagging chest colds and serious illness can keep us from our daily challenge.

But I started with the weather, so I'll stay with it a moment—that's me, practicing sticking to things.

Dealing with the elements is like dealing with so much else we can't control in life—at times inclement, at times unexpected, and at other times beautiful. Running in Tucson during the summer will be brutal most of the time, even if you get up at 5:00 AM and jump naked into your pool at the end of the run. Winter in Alaska will be unrelenting. And the rain in Portland or Seattle can be downright defeating, if we let it. But then summer in Vermont can be delicious, and winter in the California mountains can be sun-sparkle snow.

As much as we might try to take it personally, the weather is not out to get us, as in, "The universe isn't listening!" We need to deploy a lot of patience and even more grace to let go of a battle

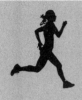

> "We need to deploy a lot of patience and even more grace to let go of a battle we simply can't win."

we simply can't win. If we don't let go, we're in danger of losing our fighting spirit for the foreseeable future. What a shame that would be, all that opportunity missed. Think like a mountain climber.

A mountaineer might spend weeks at the bottom of Mount Everest, waiting for the weather to favor her climb. That day might not come before she has to go home, which puts her out for another year. Does she give up? Of course not. She sets a new goal. She enjoys base camp. South Korean climber O Eun-Sun, who was the first woman to climb the Seven Summits (the highest peaks on seven continents), had to try more than once on many of the mountains she conquered. On Nepal's Annapurna, the last of the seven she climbed, she was forced to turn back 500 meters from the summit due to a blizzard. Five hundred meters—I can swim that in under 10 minutes. Okay, it's not quite that straightforward when the direction is up, but still. Despite what many others might see as an almost mocking defeat at the hands of Nature, O Eun-Sun simply retrenched and tackled Annapurna again, ultimately planting both feet on its peak. Climbing like a girl!

On a less daunting scale, I once flew to Montreal and then drove several hours to participate in The Canadian Ski Marathon, a two-day cross-country ski loppet, (loppet = long-distance xc ski event). Each day is an eighty-kilometer ski across a variety of terrain, including large frozen lakes, accessible only by skis in the winter.

Our plane was delayed by weather in Montreal, so we didn't arrive at our hotel until the wee hours of the morning. With only a few hours to sleep, we woke at 4:30 AM to make the bus to the 6:00 AM starting spot. When we arrived, we were hustled off the buses and bundled into a large, underheated warehouse-ish space to wait.

The same ice storm that had delayed our flight had decimated the course trails, layering on a thick, dangerously un-skiable, sheer, skating-rink surface. We waited nearly three hours, mostly huddle-squatted on the cold concrete floor, until finally the race was called off for the day. Relief mixed with disappointment, so that I barely stopped myself from crying. After all that training and travel and mental energy preparing for this day, I felt trapped at

 "The previous day's agitation evaporated within minutes of the first *shush* of my skis on the trail."

the old-world railway hotel where we were staying, too frustrated to enjoy its turn-of-the-century charm. Instead, I spent the rest of the day stewing. Now *that* was a waste of energy. The next day the grooming had managed to break the ice up enough to allow us to ski the second half of the loppet.

The previous day's agitation evaporated within minutes of the first *shush* of my skis on the trail. Who can resist nature, in all its extraordinary beauty? The crystalline trees adorned with icicles, the sharp air, and the powdery mountains glowing in the sun; the desolate frozen lakes abandoned by the summer people, and the

broad white plains, watched over by dark bony trees stripped naked by winter—the confluence of events might never happen again.
I missed a day of skiing, but I had the rare privilege of seeing a
storm-ravaged landscape seen only once in many years.

As Laurence Gonzales puts it in his fascinating book, *Deep
Survival,* "We must plan. But we must be able to let go of the plan."
The obstacles thrown up at us in our sports teach us this lesson,
again and again.

By braving the outdoors, by overcoming the challenges
Mother Nature throws at us, we reap the calming effects of being
outdoors, and discover how our athletic endeavors can literally be a
"moving meditation" for the soul. As Cherie Sank, who blogs about
her running passion, says, "There are ups and sometimes there are
downs, but mostly I'm running toward the rainbow."

We know we can't control the weather. Nature teaches us
how to deal with the unexpected setbacks to our expectations. We
can rage all we want against a rain out, or we can realign, find a new
way to live that day, to find our pleasure.

If only we could apply the same lessons weather teaches us
when we face other obstacles, such as injury. Because unlike nature,
which takes and gives simultaneously, a torn ligament or stress
fracture doesn't usually come with a haunting vista as balm for our
defeat. Injury is a risk we accept when we commit to sports.

As a cycling friend of mine once observed, "All cyclists have
either been in an accident or will be." He didn't necessarily mean
anything dramatic and horrible. He was referring to all those unexpected collisions with the pavement or trail that are bound to happen, from falling sideways after failing to unclip from your pedal,
to slipping on a rain-slicked patch of oily road (both of which I've

done), to the more serious bike accidents that leave you with broken bones. Any of which can keep you off your bike for an afternoon or six months. "Where have you had road rash?" is cycling code for, "How serious a rider are you?"

"'Where have you had road rash?' is cycling code for, 'How serious a rider are you?'"

As with cycling, so it goes in most every sport. If you have never gotten injured, I hate to break it to you, but it's probably only a matter of time. And for me that's okay; I'll take a little road rash over the potentially deleterious effects of couch potato-ism any day.

Strangely, I've found that coming back from an injury is often a reminder of how truly sweet it is to do the sport I've been missing out on, much like the seasons: I love winter partly because it doesn't last all year, and the same goes for spring, summer, and autumn. The sparkle and bite of winter giving way to the outrageous green of spring makes each more special than it could possibly be on its own. Injuries, too, are seasons in our body—a time to rest and renew. Spring will come. Our injuries will heal.

Don't get me wrong. I'm not trying to minimize injuries. I've wailed, "Why me?!" on many occasions. To no avail, of course. Ranting has yet to make me heal faster. And it doesn't change the fact that I simply can't do the sport that I want. We can rail against unfairness (remember our kind teacher the weather), or we can realign by adjusting our mind-set and activities.

Brett Buckles, a former professional ski-cross racer, struggles sometimes to adapt to the civilian life of being a "retired athlete." She was injured in a ski-cross competition in Tignes, France, when she went off a jump, twisted around backward, and flew nearly fifty feet through the air before dropping out of the sky, crushing the whole right side of her body. Miraculously, or perhaps due to her strong constitution, she healed, though she could no longer race.

"I had learned to put my all into being an elite athlete," she says. "Now it's much harder to be content with my performance in doing simple daily tasks. I am so addicted and accustomed to daily strenuous training that I don't know how to exercise in any other capacity." Still, Brett was forced to realign (or mope forever on the couch), so she found a new way of looking at the post-accident period of her life. "I now respect that my body does not need to be in perfect fitness and that it needs to relax and recover from two decades of elite training and competition."

Tanya Schine, a personal organizational consultant, had decided to turn pro when a knee injury ended her freestyle skiing. She decided to go to college instead and shifted her focus from sports for a while. Later, when she realized how much she relied on sports "to be with herself," she took up tennis and found a new arena in which to challenge herself. She's found a sport to whet her competitive appetite—tennis league tournaments. Tanya has thought a lot about what it means to her to compete. Skiing was snatched from her by an injury. She realigned. Every time she plays a game of tennis now, she asks herself, "How much am I willing to want it? If I don't win, can I handle the disappointment?"

On one occasion, Tanya was so focused on the game she was playing, on connecting her racquet to the ball, that she ran right into a cement wall. Ouch! Yet, that's the kind of focus I'd like to aim for. And the cement wall?—well, Tanya's wall was just a more concrete version of what it's like to run up against any of the obstacles life throws up in our path. Fortunately, real cement walls aside, we have the choice of crumpling at the feet of an obstacle, or bouncing off lightly, reassessing, changing direction, and seeing a new future.

Stormy weather, injury . . . enough already, well not quite. Life may also serve us up some illness and disease. I remember having one of those "worst runs ever," feeling so dragged out for no apparent reason, only to discover later the same day, as I was examining a mysterious red spot beside my ear (while simultaneously searching the web for clues as to what it might be), that I had chicken pox. The fun never stops. And there's no end to the things that might sideline us. Even the seemingly benign summer cold can throw us off course.

Erin Gish, an avid runner from California, was training for her first-ever half marathon—The Avenue of the Giants in Redwood-rich Humboldt County—when a nasty spring flu felled her. "I couldn't leave my bed for a week," she says. With only three weeks left to race day, "I couldn't imagine how I'd ever be able to complete it. I was so frustrated and discouraged, but I refused to throw in the towel. I wanted to at least show up and try, even if I had to walk half of it."

Once her fever abated, Erin began riding her bike trainer every night at a moderate intensity. With two weeks left and her cough diminished, Erin started back with short, low-intensity runs. "By that time, I had shifted my goals. I just wanted to finish. I wanted to enjoy the gorgeous setting." Realigning made all the difference. Erin finished, and while she didn't win any medals, she did enjoy the scenery.

Of course, not all illnesses are as manageable and relatively short-lived as Erin's spring flu or my bout with chicken pox. We can be struck down by diseases much less forgiving. In interviewing women for this book, I was humbled by the surprising number of women athletes who are managing chronic conditions and life-threatening diseases while pursuing their sports. We've already met Michelle Theall, and we'll meet others.

One week I happened to speak with two women who were fighting serious diseases—one had a form of stomach cancer for which she had already undergone four surgeries; and the other had Type 1 diabetes, which required a kidney transplant *and* a pancreas transplant, one year apart. I was struck by their ferocious strength and refusal to be treated as victims, or even think of themselves as such. Of course, they say they have their fair share of bad days, but they both expressed how critical it was to greet each day, "for what

 "Now, instead of focusing on winning, they take joy out of getting out on the tennis court or riding their bikes."

it was going to bring." They are both athletes, but they have changed their definitions of why they pursue their sports. Now, instead of focusing on winning, they take joy out of getting out on the tennis court or riding their bikes. Both told me how important their sports were in helping them understand how to break down challenges into achievable bite-size pieces—something critical to fighting a serious disease, which risks overwhelming the psyche if it can't be parsed.

What an apt metaphor for dealing with the inevitable pitfalls of life in general.

One day at a time.

WHEN THE PARTY IS OVER

Got a goal? Yes. Healthy and injury-free? Yes and yes. Gorgeous weather? Indeed. And yet . . .

I don't *wanna*. I punch the pillow to give it extra fluff and roll back over to sleep. In other words . . .

I've run out of gas.

I've lost heart.

My discipline is on holiday, and all the reasons I give myself for getting up and outside have left the room. The party is over and everyone fun is gone. When I turn on the lights to survey the mess, I squint against the sudden bright, too tired to face cleaning up right now.

I. Just. Can't. Do. It.

The swoosh is gone.

Welcome to burnout. This is when training becomes a tedious exercise in going from one race to the next, or one training day to the next, until we ask ourselves, "Why? What's the point? Who really cares anyway?" We are exhausted, in the most literal sense of the word, as in depleted and empty—psychologically and physically. We have just plain worn ourselves out pursuing our ambitions.

Among psychologists, sports burnout is variously defined as "a psychological, emotional, and physical withdrawal from a formerly pursued and enjoyable sport as a result of excessive stress which acts on the athlete over time," or "the manifestation or consequence of the situational, cognitive, physiologic, and behavioral components of excessive stress."

"Some days (really, some months) we're just not feeling it."

Stress. Stress. Stress. We can't overtax our bodies, in the same way we can't overtax ourselves at work, or with a jam-packed social life. Our body needs a vacation from its routines. Our mind needs a break from the discipline of the daily challenge.

As exercise physiologists are quick to point out, more is not always better. We need to listen to our bodies. Some days (really, some months) we're just not feeling it. And that's perfectly natural. So long as we hear the message our body is sending us. If we ignore the time-to-slow-down warning, we risk more serious consequences—critical depletions of B6, causing an aggravated form of anemia; vital exhaustion, forcing months of rest; and injuries, such as stress fractures, which are notorious overtraining messages.

On the tennis court, Tanya has worked hard to find the right balance of frequency, maintaining and improving her game, and not getting worn out on the sport. To that end, she has also tried to find the balance between tournament play, where a bad game means you're out, which she finds can be too stressful; and league tennis, which, though it lacks the "rush" of tournaments, is more fun and still fuels her competitive zeal. She has realized that playing tennis three times a week is great, but that playing four or five times a week doesn't make her a better player. In fact, it can have a deleterious effect, sapping her energy and leading to injury, which can be burnout's way of saying, "Hi there, time for a break."

When Tanya was finally laid off from tennis with a shoulder and elbow injury from overuse, she reevaluated again. She thinks that when she gets back to tennis she'll return to the rush of tournaments. "I might lose, but I'll still have a good time." Why? Because what fuels our spirit changes over time and the trick to not burning out is to recognize those inflection points, as Tanya has, and stay fresh in our approach.

 "The worst part of burnout is that we run out of *enthusiasm* for our sport."

The worst part of burnout isn't that we start to underachieve because we lack the energy to achieve at the level we've set for ourselves. No. The worst part of burnout is that we run out of *enthusiasm* for our sport. We lose track of the fun, and "fun" is the *why* of it all. Why do anything if there's no element of pleasure. I admit it. I'm a hedonist at core. And my training is part of that hedonism. I do the sports I do because they are a profound source of enjoyment.

Nora stopped figure skating when she went to college and it was clear that the oft-dreamed-of Olympics were not in her future. She couldn't go back to the rink for ten years. *Ten years.* To a place she'd been going almost every day for most of her life. For so long she had defined herself by skating that she needed time before she could be on the ice without feeling like she needed to be taking skating as seriously as possible. She had burned the fun out, at least temporarily. Now, more than a decade later, she's found new sports—triathlons, marathons, hiking, rock climbing, yoga, and more. And in the winter, she likes to spend the odd afternoon skating peacefully with her husband in the outdoor rink at the park.

There are two things we can do to avoid burnout. First we need to rest. No, I mean *really* rest, as in legs up, body relaxed, eating bonbons, preferably served by someone lovely in your life, surrounded by fluffy pillows; or on a deck chair with the breeze gently blowing, frozen or up, the drink choice is yours. Second—we must change our routine. You may have heard the expression "A change is as good as a rest," but have you tried it lately?

That could very well be Rebecca Rusch's motto.

The world champion adventure racer gave me new insight into how to avoid burnout. Rebecca does not come by her athleticism naturally. In fact, no one else in her family is the least athletic, and quite a few of them weigh in higher on the scale than is healthy. As a teen, she worried about getting fat. In high school, a friend suggested they join the cross-country running team. "You'll never get fat," she said, "and you'll get a free sweat suit." Rebecca thought both those things sounded like a pretty solid idea, so she joined.

Well she hasn't gotten fat, that's for sure. And now she makes her living as an athlete. But not as a distance runner. In fact, Rebecca has picked up a whole variety of other athletic pursuits. First she devoured rock climbing. It's still her first love, so much so that she owned her own rock gym and led guided climbs for other enthusiasts. Then she competed as a member of the U.S. Women's Whitewater Rafting Team before shifting next into adventure racing, where she maintains her "champion athlete" status. To top it all off, she also picked up mountain biking.

I'd add that she's also a champion at avoiding burnout.

Rebecca's willingness to reinvent herself, to begin again in a new sport, allows her to maintain fluidity in her sports identity, which has helped her avoid getting burned out.

That's a rare trait. We like to hang on to our identities. We become attached to who we are. For example, "I'm a first-thing-in-the-morning workout person," or "I'm the kind of person who packs for a trip at the last minute."

When we are attached to our identity, we begin to measure ourselves in the same way. Every challenge is one we've seen before. We develop expectations of ourselves. Do you always do 5ks or marathons? Do you always do century bike rides? Or ski over moguls instead of cross-country? Have you always pursued jobs as a lawyer in a law firm? Why not a nonprofit? And what about the men you date? Must they all be over six feet tall? There's nothing wrong with sameness, but sometimes it's good to change things up.

Yes, to be strong healthy women we need to identify ourselves as such. But we need to be careful, too, not to set that identity in stone or we risk becoming confined to a narrow prison instead of feeling free to define ourselves with new richness every day. Just as we cannot become overly attached to our goals, so it is with our identity. "I am a runner" can become a too-confining identity if you develop an injury that prevents you from running. Instead, we can find another way to be strong while our injury heals.

> "After all, it can be downright *joyful* to discover a new passion, to discover, even, that you're incredibly good at it."

Identity is about possibility, not about strictures. One of the bonuses of keeping our identity fluid is that it enables us to see ourselves in new ways. Instead of always measuring our accomplishments by the same narrow standards, ask yourself the following question: What am I capable of? This isn't a historical research question, although it's good to draw insight from past accomplishments. Rather, it is a question aimed at the future. As in, "What *could* I be capable of, if I tried?"

After all, it can be downright *joyful* to discover a new passion, to discover, even, that you're incredibly good at it. By doing so, you avoid the disillusionment, boredom, and burnout that can come from measuring yourself by the same standards in the same sport, year after year. After all, "begin" and "burn out" together are an oxymoron. The expression is not "The weariness of the beginner." Rather, it is "The *enthusiasm* of a beginner."

Which brings me back to the yogic notion of tapas. In his book, Kraftsow points out that tapas is about breaking cycles of habit and addiction. It's about shifting the momentum of our daily lives so that we are more actively aware of why we are doing what we are doing (whether it's going to soccer practice, dating someone new, or eating a piece of rhubarb pie) and whether it enhances our life. It encourages us to see things in a new way. Applied to sports, if our routine becomes so entrenched that it degrades us physically, mentally, or emotionally, then our daily discipline—our tapas—has become warped instead of helping us to be more present in our lives. And that's exactly what burnout is, the point at which our sport, our workouts, become so habitual that we fail to see the point at which they no longer serve us.

Eckhart Tolle, in his book *The Power of Now*, suggests we take time each day to "flood our body with consciousness." By which he means to literally close our eyes, lie quietly, and focus our attention on each part of our body until we can *feel* it as a single field of energy. That's being in the moment. There's no doubt that if we pay close attention to our bodies, they will tell us what's best. And sometimes that's "stay the course," or "rev up," and other times the message is "change now."

It can be liberating to begin again, to *not* be the expert, with all its associated expectations. Take away the measuring stick every once in a while. Remind yourself of what being a child feels like, to thrill in your own ability, to feel awe. Awe at the world, yes, but awe in the face of your own capacity to renew your life.

GETTING OUR DAILY DOSE OF THE INEFFABLE

Once, after I had struggled through an off day in a fifty-kilometer cross-country ski loppet, a friend asked me why I did it. The race was hard and it was lonely. The narrative in my head was a babble of "Keep going, you can do it" and "Are you crazy? Give it up. You started cross-country skiing way too late in life. You'll never finish." The race wasn't pretty. I may well have been the last person to cross the line, my technique in a shambles, but it was glorious nonetheless. That loppet wasn't the first time and it won't be the last time I finish bottom of the pack.

"Wow," a friend of mine once commented to me after a different, but equally long, cross-country skiing race, "DFL, that's impressive."

DFL—Dead Fucking Last—it's not necessarily an acronym you want applied to yourself.

And yet, why do I do it?

For that feeling of exhaustion so profound even my shins are tingling from the exertion; more, for the privilege nature bestows on me of her quiet, magnificent beauty. And for the reward of facing down the negative narrative in my head, which is so deeply delightful. Each time I prove to myself that I can do *it*, I get a little buzz of pride, and that makes the next challenge (in sports or elsewhere) all that much easier. Every day that I get out of bed and make it out onto the road, into the snow, the pool, or the yoga studio, I've not only overcome another challenge, I am reestablishing my place in the world. I am reminding myself of what possibility means.

Becky Salmon knows what I'm talking about. A small business owner and passionate swimmer, Becky has an eye condition called "strabismus," which means her eyes work independently of one another. Although she's undergone a variety of different therapies, she often sees double and has been wearing bifocals since the age of twenty. Her depth perception is way off, and she has headaches more days than she doesn't. But in college, Becky found a new friend in swimming. She had decided to do a triathlon, but

 "To her amazement, she discovered that water was her superhero suit, her x-ray vision."

the catch was that she needed to learn how to swim. To her amazement, she discovered that water was her superhero suit, her x-ray vision. "Other than when I'm sleeping, swimming is literally the only time I can rest my eyes," Becky says. "It's a total release."

Empowered, Becky zoomed past the usual swimming goals and dove into competitive long-distance swimming. "My first 'real' long-distance open-water swim was off Saint Croix—five miles in the open ocean. We were ferried out on boats to Buck Island Reef, which makes you realize how far it's really going to be. Was I nervous!"

With only about one hundred swimmers, when the conch shell blows it's easy to feel alone pretty quickly. "After about five hundred yards the ocean floor drops away," says Becky. "I was awestruck by the sparkling starfish hanging above the bottomless, dark blue sea. They looked like constellations."

I was envious when she described this world upside down, the sky in the sea.

Her next thought was, "I'm good. I can do this!" She did. And she went on to do it several more times, even getting stung by a Portuguese man–of–war once. "It caused excruciating, searing pain . . ." she says. Did it stop her? Of course not. She had found her ineffable, her reason to get in the water almost every day.

Every *day?* Sound daunting? Nope. We're up for it.

On a recent chill morning, it took all my Susan B. Anthony "hardihood of spirit" just to put on my running shoes. All night I'd listened to the low whistle of the wind through the windows. I knew the air by the river would feel ten degrees colder than what the thermometer promised.

Did I really need to do this?

Today? *Again?*

Nope. I didn't. But I pushed myself out the door anyway.

Dawn was creeping slowly into the sky. The moon hung over the gray Hudson River, roiling in the wind. Five and half miles upriver, the George Washington Bridge (my destination and the turnaround point of my run) adorned the horizon like a jeweled necklace, its lights winking in the wan morning sky. My head refused to join me on the run, letting my cold-stiffened legs slog slowly north without benefit of mental support. When I reached the bridge, I ran out to the little red lighthouse of storybook fame, as I always do. Just to say hello to the small structure, so overshadowed by the gargantuan majesty of the bridge looming over it. For some reason, I lifted my gaze more than usual and looked out past the lighthouse, up the Hudson. The Palisades cliffs glowed a pale orange, brushed by the light of the newly risen winter sun. The river snaked north, flowing around a bend, continuing its journey out of my sight. I felt the pull of the unknown, the possibility of a journey upriver, watched over by the benevolent cliffs rising up from the riverbanks. I turned south again and headed home, my heart light, having had my daily dose of the ineffable.

CHAPTER 4:

The Goldilocks Principle

"Strive for moderation in all you do . . . In this way you use the balancing tendency of the current forces to center yourself."
—I Ching no. 15

I t's my first day of the season on cross-country skis, and I stumble on the soft snow, clacking my skis together as I jerk-glide up the steep-ish hill. This is supposed to be a silent sport, but instead I sound like a percussion section with no rhythm. I flap my poles in an ineffectual, reflexive attempt to balance myself, and for a second I wonder if, with my flailing arms, I might levitate above the earth's surface, on which today it seems a challenge to even stay upright. Isn't there an age past which I will no longer fall flat on my face? And I don't mean metaphorically, though that would be nice, too. Within minutes I'm shaking with exhaustion. Wasn't I fit just yesterday? Was this same ascent so endless last year?

Then suddenly I'm at the top. I look down onto the valley below, the soft white snow dunes dotted with occasional dark green groves of pine trees. The thin air is sharp on my lungs, though in a couple of days I know I'll be used to the altitude again. I stop caring that I apparently can't ski anymore. Then, just when I've let go of any expectation, I find my feet planted firmly on my skis, and we remember each other, my skis and me, and how well we fit together. Then I *do* fly, down the hill, with arms outstretched, balanced beautifully and improbably on two thin strips of colorfully painted carbon fiber, heart singing.

B alance is a delicate thing. Often we think of balance as something hard and fixed. Balance doesn't work that way; rather, it is a dynamic process, constantly shifting.

We know this physically. When we are standing still, *feeling* balanced, our body is actually keeping itself upright by making thousands of tiny micro-adjustments: our feet replanted in the earth, the shift and sway of our ankles and knees indiscernible to the naked eye. Our hips above our knees, supporting our core, the muscles of which engage to fight gravity, keeping our backs upright; and so on up to our heavy bobble head, which threatens to topple us with its disproportionate weight. If our bodies weren't in constant motion, we would literally fall over.

There's really no difference between finding physical balance and finding any other kind of balance in our lives, whether it's psychological, emotional, spiritual, social, professional . . . you get the picture. Finding our personal fulcrum is a dynamic endeavor. Just like with our bodies, if our lives are out of balance, we, too, will metaphorically fall over.

Dubbed "America's Life Balance Expert" by the media, Ed Mc-Donough says, "Stress, anxiety, information overload, and countless expectations set upon you . . . can easily throw your body, mind, and spirit into a state of imbalance, and your life into a state of disarray."

In the stories of the life of the Buddha, this disarray is described musically. Buddha is said to have discovered The Middle Path (an essential principle of Buddhism, which is finding balance between extremes) when he heard a fisherman playing a stringed instrument and realized that the music could not be as beautiful if one of the strings were too loose, or indeed too tight. We are all fishermen and our lives are our instrument. Too much of one thing or not enough of another will result in disharmony.

To find balance is to find our best path in life—The Middle Path.

How do we find balance? And why do we lose it to begin with?

WE ALL WALK OUR OWN TIGHTROPES

When we close our eyes and think of balance, we might first smell the dust and hay floor and the hot rubberized canvas of the circus big top. High up, the tightrope is already suspended, titillating us with its promise. For me, balance also calls to mind the film image of 1970s French high wire artist Philippe Petit, who was immortalized in the 2008 documentary *Man on Wire*, as he skips lightly between the two towers of the World Trade Center.

One of my early experiences with balance was on a tight-rope as well, or at least a sort-of-one. I was ten or so, and a friend I often played with after school instituted "circus practice" for us. She declared that we would "learn to walk the tightrope." She also promised me that her father, who was no more than a shadowy figure to me, would bring us the special "sticky shoes" that all the professionals used, just as soon as he got home from wherever he was. We began our training on a long two-by-four placed precariously (I now realize) across two sawhorses. At first I had to shore up my courage before the first step onto the plank, going through what I thought was proper tightrope procedure: straightening my shoulders, standing on one foot and then the other, until, with a deep breath and a bit of a flutter in my belly, I'd point one toe and slowly slide one foot in front of the other out onto the plank. But after only a few practices, the zing of fear was gone, replaced by a certain boredom. The plank was wide and even when it flipped up behind us like a teeter-totter, as it was wont to do at times, the

"There have been times in life when I've longed for the equivalent of sticky shoes, that magic something to keep me balanced when life feels helter-skelter."

ground was so near we could jump down easily. Our practices fell on hard times when I began to wonder where the sticky shoes were, without which we couldn't progress to a real rope, tied, I hoped, between the branches of two tall trees. In the end, I didn't have the chance to find out, because my friend moved away before the next school year began, and at that age, it didn't occur to me to question whether such shoes existed in the first place.

There have been times in life when I've longed for the equivalent of sticky shoes, that magic something to keep me balanced when life feels helter-skelter. Is this marriage really not meant to last forever? Can I forge a new career? Will I make friends in this unfamiliar place? Do I have what it takes to finish the training for the long race I've signed up for?

There are no sticky shoes. There is only us, finding our footing anew this year, this month, or even just today.

What, exactly, is this thing called balance anyway?

Here are some of the beautiful words that define it in all its variety: "equilibrium, even, harmony, poise, sanity, steady. . . ." The words are evocative, expressing the fluidity of the concept. There's no one and only way to achieve balance; just as the sum of eight can be arrived at in a myriad of ways other than four plus four.

We all walk our own tightropes, sometimes easily, and at other times with great difficulty.

Finding the correct balance between work and play, stillness and activity, family time and personal time, puts us on the road to a more harmonious life.

The first time I met the *idea* of balance in life may have been from reading Goldilocks and the Three Bears, about a little girl who wants things "just right": porridge that is neither too hot nor too cold; a bed that is neither too hard nor too soft.

Scientists have appropriated the story for their own purposes, using the Goldilocks Principle to describe things in nature that, to exist or to function effectively, must fall within certain parameters that do not veer to extremes. Human beings, for example, live on a Goldilocks planet—not too close and not too far from the sun, but *just right*. A little off one way or the other, and life as we know it would not exist. Of course, the Goldilocks Principle assumes that humans behave in a way that maintains nature's equilibrium as well, something we seem to be doing a poor job of (but I'll leave that to Al Gore and others more versed in the topic to extrapolate on). Everything has to be "just right" for our natural environment to function at its best. Remove an important element from nature's intricate web, like our ozone layer, and it falls to pieces, creating a cascade effect of damage. Out of balance, our ecosystem collapses.

As in nature, we need to maintain balance within the areas of our life or we risk having them collapse as well. Fortunately, it turns out that finding the balance *between* the different parts of our life helps bring balance to the individual parts of our life and to our life in general.

A survey conducted by the National Athlete Career and Education program (ACE) and the Australian Institute of Sport (AIS) asked athletes about the integration of sports into their lives. In response to questions about the role education has played in achieving a balanced lifestyle, they variously said, "[Education] puts sport in perspective," and "It gives me the ability to be a whole person . . . I am able to focus on different aspects of my life. Therefore I do not burn out or over focus and lose sight of the big picture."

And from a different "outback," Nora Hunt, a sports counselor and former top rodeo athlete, wrote on the website Pretty Tough, "I don't believe that you can compete at your highest level if your personal life is unbalanced. The way we perform is a reflection of our everyday lives, so managing and constantly learning to prioritize what is important is essential if we want to achieve peak performance."

For Renee Hesker, being the full-time mother of two young children, it's her morning workout that helps focus the rest of her day and grants her precious moments of "Renee time" before she plunges into the demands of caregiving. "Without the athletic outlet, it's hard for me to feel fully there."

Shifting to our sports can release us from being overly focused on stress that is related to work, family, or relationships, often providing us the distance needed to gain a fresh perspective or even just shed the detritus of the day.

Rebecca, the tire-changing whiz from Texas, puts it this way. "Sports are almost like purification for me. Every bad thing is taken away, the pizza I might have had the night before, the stress and anger from an argument, or just the frustration from work. I become my favorite person all over again; the one who is not worried about what she looks like or how others see her; the one who is a strong determined fighter." Personally, I have solved more problems during the course of a workout and answered more questions that have been plaguing me than I can count. There have been moments I've wanted to leap up off the yoga mat and call someone with an idea. During runs I have wished for pen and paper. Instead I'll recite the burst of insight to myself like a mantra until I'm sure it's embedded enough into my short-term memory that I'll be able to recall it when I get home.

Lisa Barnes, a runner and triathlete, wrote the following blog post on her Spinster Chronicles about finding balance after she broke off her engagement and was plunged into the sometimes harsh world of being a single woman in her thirties, in a society that prizes marriage:

 "Am I a runner? Or just a broken heart with Nikes . . ."

*Am I a runner? Or just a broken heart with Nikes . . .
Are you a runner when you have to run to feel less
insane? If the adrenaline that you feel from a run
sedates you enough so that you can rationalize your
feelings and restore a sense of calmness in your life,
are you running? Or are you drugging yourself with
endorphins? If I didn't have a release from the "What
Ifs?" and "Why hasn't hes?" I am sure that I would
be in a padded room somewhere chanting, "I'll never
tell . . . " I have accepted realities, admitted faults,
forgiven and forgotten over years and miles. There are
no secrets from myself when I run. I can't choose what
I will think about or what conflicts I will acknowledge
when I go for a run, but one thing that is guaranteed is
that I will have to confront them.*

Like Lisa, I find that when I have the space and time to let
things really come up, then I better pave the way for letting them
go. Then, what do you know, I seem to have more room to be happy. That's balancing and rebalancing.

Nora Frank, the former competitive figure skater, was for
years ultra-dedicated to her skating. It was the center of her life.
She was young and skating seemed like "everything" to her. When
she realized that skating could not be her whole life, she gave up
the sport completely. Skating was all or nothing for Nora. She
needed to rebalance. Now she gets out almost every day on her
bike, in the pool, or on the mountain, but sports are a way to off-
set the demands of her career, to provide an opportunity to shift
her focus.

"It's an issue of control. When I have my workout plan, it feels peaceful and powerful. I literally feel like I would *look* different if I didn't work out in the morning," she says.

I can relate. For me it's that I feel cleaner after my shower on the days that I sweat. A shower on a rest day is not nearly as satisfying. Even when I'm physically fatigued and know I need to rest my body, it's sometimes hard for me to luxuriate in the day off. But I know it's part of maintaining balance, and without the rest, I'll be drawing a "go-to-jail" card soon enough and will be *forced* to take time off.

WE ALREADY HAVE OUR STICKY SHOES

So how do we *find* our balance? For starters, balance is a custom fit that's different for everyone. No one can really tell us *what* our individual balance should look like. It's up to us to decide if 25 percent of our free time should be dedicated to surfing the web or doing yoga or training for a triathlon or catching up on lost sleep. Balance is really a case of "we know it when we feel it." Like the physical sensation of falling, our internal sensors tell us when we're off balance—dragging through a workout, a fight with your spouse about . . . what was it about? or an outbreak of psoriasis are all good indicators of something awry. So, too, we can sense when our life is in harmony.

"Like the physical sensation of falling, our internal sensors tell us when we're off balance. . . . "

One of the ways we can more reliably achieve equilibrium is by literally practicing how to balance physically. Remember, who we are is how we move. The idea applies to balance.

For example, if I can find my balance in yoga, then I am better equipped to find my balance in the world. If I haven't practiced balance in yoga (or in another discipline), then when I chance to find a moment of balance elsewhere in the world, it will be quite by accident. Until we understand things explicitly, until we surface things to our consciousness, they are not readily accessible to us when we need them—on demand, as it were. That is the work of practice, or training, in sports as it is in life.

"The unique connection between mind and body is essential to achieving any goal," says Nora, the sports counselor we met above. "For example, if you want to adapt better in pressure situations, then work on becoming more flexible both mentally and physically. Take a deep breath and practice 'going with the flow.' Physically, you can adopt a stretching or yoga practice into your workout schedule. Training yourself mentally and physically will help you deal with stressful or difficult circumstances." Balance is *not* stressful. Have you ever noticed how easeful good physical balance feels? How effortless it feels when we find that sweet spot where all the wobbly stops and we could stand on one leg forever. No sticky shoes required. Balance is not about force. It's not about pushing or pulling, or muscling aside imbalance. We can't squeeze in that extra hour of workout at the expense of precious sleep and think we'll get away with being unfocused and cantankerous with everyone at work the next day. Our work performance will slip. Our colleagues will grow tired of our crankiness. Balance is finding that combination of energy and gentle stillness that enables us to function at our best, to get the most out of our lives.

In other words, balance is a happy place.

And that's the place we want to be. Today.

So balance also takes us back to how we approach the daily challenge. Yes, sports are about being, as our flight attendant friend Lois says, a "moving kind of girl," but it is also about stillness, about *rest*.

One of my yoga instructors who teaches Yin Yoga, a branch that focuses on poses held for three to five minutes, says, "You're done with the doing, doing, doing part of your day. Now is the time when you practice *not* doing."

"We are experts at doing too much, at overtaxing ourselves."

Holding a yoga pose for five minutes can seem like an eternity. But as my instructor points out, we have no problem filling our lives up. We are experts at doing too much, at overtaxing ourselves. The challenge is figuring out where and how not to fill our lives up too much. For most of us, finding the moments to soften is infinitely more difficult than pushing harder. To accomplish things, to achieve our goals, we need to also learn how to let go of the need to accomplish.

Sounds counterintuitive, but it's not. We can feel the truth of this in our bodies. When I am *trying* to come into physical balance, I often struggle to find the right stance. The days I don't struggle, the days I don't grumble to myself, "I'm going to get this balance or else," are usually the days that balance comes like a sigh, an easy release from one moment to the next, because I'm not facing off with my goal of balancing. Instead I'm taking what comes my way.

"It's only yoga," says another of my yoga instructors, when she senses that the class is getting frustrated by an advanced pose. By the same token, it's only a workout, it's only a race, it's only. . . . If we want to take things seriously, we also need to take them lightly. Attachment to an outcome stiffens us. Balance is supple.

Balance implies taking a little of this and giving a little of that. Sometimes balance takes a little, or asks us to give a little, whether we want to or not.

Laural Ringler, an adventure mentor for families, teens, individuals, and groups, had to give up soccer, a sport she adored, after sustaining a serious ankle injury. "I had to work hard to remind myself that 'it's only soccer,' to get my head around it," she says. "I didn't tell anyone for a while. I didn't want to give it up. But when I weighed all the other athletic activities I wanted to be doing—hiking, bicycling, a little triathlon here and there—against the 'can't-do-because-of-injuries-from-soccer,' it seemed ludicrous to continue."

"As with any first love, I am nostalgic for the fluid moments of soccer," she continues. "I won't stop being active, but I'm changed, and so are my options."

In Gro Hart's case, life circumstances enforce a balance. The forty-something nationally ranked amateur triathlete is the parent of an autistic child, so her training is a major source of stress relief, a much-needed escape, and something she gets to do just for her. She competes hard and it pays off. "It takes so much just to get to the starting line with all there is to manage at home, I'm damned if I'm not going to have the best race I can."

Yet the challenges of her life at home are built-in obsession prevention. She's forced by the demands of the rest of her life to keep everything in perspective. She's always calm before a race because in the context of the rest of her life, it is only a race.

We learn how to feel balance with our bodies, to inhabit the sensation of poise, and that knowledge spreads to the rest of our lives. In our relationship with sports, that means knowing when to go hard and when to ease up. In fact, that's pretty much what it means in everything else we do, too.

But there's a catch. No one else can give you the exact recipe for achieving your personal balance.

ONE GIRL'S *"AHHHH"* IS ANOTHER GIRL'S *"UGH"*

The pursuit of happiness is highly individual, and therefore so is the definition of balance. For me, there is an enormous reward to be gained in pushing myself beyond what I thought was my limit. Yet pushing beyond the limit *sounds* unbalanced—until we remember that balance does not equal limit. Balance, as we've seen, is an agile concept, constantly adjusting to new circumstances. True, to find balance is to know our boundaries or comfort zones (as in—I'm not up for that seven-hour mountain marathon right now. With the various work and home obligations I need to attend to right now, the training just wouldn't fit in); which is very different from setting limits (as in—I could never do that seven-hour marathon, it would be way too hard for me).

Kristy, who plays on the U.S. Women's Bandy Team, puts it this way, "To others, my balance may seem different because my priorities are different. My balance comes with 'have I recently spent time with those I love?' If I answer 'no,' I know that I have crossed the line and I need to step back some."

For me, the test is always this—are my sports diminishing my ability to enjoy all the other things in life that are important to me? For example, if I'm too tired from working out to go to the movies (a passion of mine), or I have no time left to read (another passion), or my training schedule is so rigorous that there's no room for a long evening with friends overflowing with conversation (ditto on the passion), then I feel like I'm losing my way. It's a fine line, and where that line is drawn for me is not the same as where it is for others.

Like happiness, balance is not an absolute concept. There is no perfect happiness, nor is there perfect balance. Perfection, or at least as we commonly think of it, is a confining concept, one that holds up a rigid ideal as a benchmark for all of us. But what of the pursuit of "excellence" over perfection? It is a concept that better captures the ideal of balance, because it represents room for variability. My "excellent" marathon time is someone else's bad day, which takes nothing away from my own accomplishment. Excellence is putting in our best effort and holding ourselves to our own highest standard; which is far different from perfection, that more

"Excellence is putting in our best effort and holding ourselves to our own highest standard. . . . "

confining concept, which implies the best of the best of the best, as defined by the whole world—the perfect Olympic ski jump, the perfect gymnastics routine, a perfect score on the LSATs.

As Carl Jung said, "Perfection belongs to the gods; the most that we can hope for is excellence." What a wonderful pursuit.

Mary Beth Gonzales found her own "excellent balance" by combining her love of sports with her career as a certified public accountant. Mary Beth is one of those rare women who can say, with truth, that she's played sports literally all of her life. She began with soccer at two years old and never looked back—basketball, volleyball, soccer, marathons, and fitness competitions. Sports were as essential to her as eating, and while she found ways to balance her athletic pursuits with her career, her dream of life balance was to fuse the two.

While working as an accountant, she earned her personal training certification, spent a year attending conferences in the field, and experienced an epiphany: AlaVie Fitness, a fitness business. By hooking her financial brain up with her personal training proclivities and skills, she finessed the framework of a fitness community that offered outdoor boot camps primarily for women, and provided a network of health and wellness professionals available to members.

"The biggest thing I didn't expect when I started the business was the relationships people build through the programs," says Mary Beth. "Not all women have the flexibility to join a soccer team to get their workouts in, and it helps to have a source of team spirit and motivation to get them and keep them in shape. That's what's behind AlaVie."

You could almost call Mary Beth, a kind of "sports yenta," or matchmaker, for friendships. Now that's got to be fulfilling.

What fills *you* up? What provides you the pleasure and privilege of being connected to something you enjoy? It might be sports or books or movies or naps; it could be cooking or writing or gardening or belly dancing. It's different for all of us. One woman's *"ahhhh"* could be another woman's *"ugh!"*

Filled up. Full. Ful-filled. But remember, "filled up" is not the same thing as "overflowing." The art of being full is finding the "just right" combination in everything we do. And by focusing on our self, by finding "just right," we can make those around us feel pretty alright, too.

SELF-*CENTERED* IS NOT SELFISH

What's good for the goose is good for the gander, and the homily applies equally in our sports. Staying in shape, rejuvenating ourselves through playing sports, is *good* for us, and when it's not shortchanging the people in our lives, from family and friends, to our employers—it's more than likely good for *them*, too.

Sure, on the surface, spending hours running, swimming, cycling, or kicking a ball around a field can *seem* like selfish pursuits in an already busy life, but we're not the only beneficiaries. In addition to being happier, less stressed people, we're also more productive and motivated employees and colleagues, and data proves we're also much healthier, which means we cost less in the healthcare system. In other words, we're an asset when we run like a girl; when we are in balance, there is nothing selfish about being active.

Heidi, the social worker and avid marathoner from New York who pointed out the dearth of X chromosomes in the sports pages, works in the criminal justice system. Her job is all about giving—a lot—to others, every day. "Taking care of myself is non-negotiable. I am no good to anyone if I haven't been good to myself."

Indeed. It's hard to help others be happy and whole if we aren't. For Heidi, getting in some kind of exercise—whether it's a run or some time at the gym—is like sleep. "You need to know yourself and your own needs," she says. "That's not selfish, it's self-awareness."

What does the word "selfish" mean anyway? I'll tell you: it's eating all the leftover chocolate cake without asking *me* if I wanted some, even though you *knew* that I would, but you didn't ask because that would mean less for you. Grrrr.

Merriam-Webster defines selfish as to be "concerned excessively or exclusively with oneself; seeking or concentrating on one's own advantage, pleasure, or well-being without regard for others."

Taking care of ourselves, even to put ourselves first, is a not bad thing. The key words here are "excessive," "exclusive," and "without regard for others." When we're approaching our sports in a balanced way, we are not selfish, we are "centered" on our self to be more centered for others.

To prioritize our needs is not selfish. The airlines have it right: put on your own oxygen mask first. If we're not breathing, how are we going to help those next to us?

When we are empty, we have nothing to give. When we are full ourselves, we will find that we have a deep well of love, energy,

"The airlines have it right: put on your own oxygen mask first."

and time to give to others, those close to us, and even strangers. That's Heidi's point.

Pursuing things for our "self" is not selfish unless in doing so we disregard someone else's needs. For example, if I set the alarm for 5:00 AM on my workout days, but on my days off, I have a fit if my partner sets the alarm early because it will interfere with my sleep—never mind that I've interfered with *his* sleep all week—that's selfish. Our needs may come first for us, but part of balance is adjusting how we fulfill our needs so that they don't actively interfere with other people's needs, particularly those close to us who are most affected by our behavior and activities.

Katie Morgan, a thirty-something triathlete who works in the insurance business, describes her intense commitment to training as "self-serving." Katie does Ironman races, and has also done the grueling *Marathon des Sables*, six days of endurance running across the Sahara Desert in Morocco. Her first Ironman was a "rebound relationship" after a bad breakup, so in a sense the race was, as she puts it, "all about me." But does that make her Ironman selfish? No. It makes her centered. And as you'll see, cultivating strength in the face of deep emotional pain has always been her go-to therapy.

Just before Katie graduated from high school, her mother died of cancer. To lose a mother is heartbreaking enough, but Katie also had to endure seeing her mother suffer through her illness for years, overshadowing most of Katie's teen years (as if those years aren't difficult enough for most of us). She recalls one occasion where she even went with her mother and father to look at a burial plot. That doesn't leave a lot of room for being an adolescent. For years after her mother's death, Katie charged ahead, carrying out the plan her mother had laid out for her before she died, which included going to college. She rushed off to Penn State just months after her mother died, but she found that when she'd come home during holidays, she felt a growing envy of her younger sister and brother, of their free-spirited play in the yard. Of being *children*. She had missed out on that.

 "[S]he felt a growing envy of her younger sister and brother, of their free-spirited play in the yard. Of being *children*."

For Katie, running, biking, and swimming *are* play; it's her way of getting back the joy she lost in adolescence. In fact, Katie recently got into a new relationship, and she's going through a period of *re*balancing to fit him into her life, which is pretty solid insurance against obsession. It's all about *happy*.

So when does balance disintegrate into obsession?

Jodi, the musher from Alaska, is sometimes kidded by friends that her "addiction" to mushing is more expensive than a cocaine habit. Jodi says that while her sport may seem like obsession to some, "The life I lead is the best one I could ask for." And mushing is a hugely demanding winter sport. One year, Jodi was so busy with her dogs and racing, she didn't have time for Christmas. She sent out an email to family and friends and told them that she'd decided to celebrate Christmas in April. So her family enjoyed a "second" belated holiday celebration with Jodi; after all, exchanging a few presents, whatever the month, never goes amiss.

Staying healthy and connected to others while also being centered on ourselves is a pretty good measure against obsession. But if instead our athletic pursuits blind us to the rest of our lives, there's a good chance we're slithering dangerously down into the pit of obsession.

CLEATS ARE A MUST FOR SLIPPERY SLOPES

Obsessed? Who *me*?

The thin line between just enough and too much is different for everyone.

Sports can widen the margins of our lives, literally taking us to new places on our feet, our bikes, hanging from ropes, or in a boat. And they can metaphorically take us to new places in our minds, showing us possibility we never knew existed before.

Or, sports can become the horse-blinders of obsession.

Getting injured, feeling exhausted, losing touch with relationships—it might be time to review our priorities.

Donna Elliot, who for years balanced an active career with caving, rock climbing, and mountain climbing, says it's a red flag that you're obsessed when "it starts to damage personal relationships, affect your job, or results in too many injuries."

Or as Kelly, the coach and professional triathlete says, "It's not so much 'obsessed,' as it is 'constantly dedicated.' I have always been a busybody like my dad." Her husband points out that even if she stopped competing seriously in triathlons, she'd still "go hard."

Kelly is simply one of those people who is hardwired to seek out challenges. Pushing herself *is* Kelly's version of balance.

I can relate because I thrive on challenge, too. But the slope gets slippery when dedication interferes with the rest of our lives, when challenges overwhelm us.

It helps to have cleats on the slippery slope of obsession. We can don them ourselves—by keeping tabs on whether we are maintaining balance in our lives. Or, our metaphoric cleats can be forced upon us by circumstances, good and bad—work and family obligations, injuries and illness. Because obsession unchecked can keep sliding down that slippery slope into addiction. Sports, it turns out, can be our cleats against addiction.

Addiction. Just the word makes me want to cover my eyes with my hands, which I tend to do when I'm watching a film of someone shooting up heroin. Right now I'm thinking of Harvey Keitel in *The Bad Lieutenant.*

On its face, addiction just sounds all-around *bad.* When really, addictions run the gamut, and some aren't all that damaging. Addiction happens when we hook into our pleasure center, when that dopamine rush gets a grip on us and we're helpless in its grasp. Really though, how evil is chocolate?

When we're "hooked" on something that so jazzes us up, at times we think we can't live without it—or him . . . or her. We like to say we're "addicted to" this or that, but really it's more about getting our quick fix, a little zing of pleasure. Me, I get my fix through chocolate, Bob's Red Mill dried blueberries, the occasional diet

"We like to say we're 'addicted to' this or that, but really it's more about getting our quick fix, a little zing of pleasure."

coke, movies, and, of course, running up steep rocky mountains in pursuit of expansive views. For others, it might be the *Daily Show with Jon Stewart*, walking the dog at sunset, fresh-cut pineapple, or a sunset paddle in the kayak. Unfortunately, as we move along the spectrum, our fixes can become destructive and damaging addictions: buying and hoarding expensive designer shoes we can't afford, having unprotected sex with strangers, smoking, or heroin. And as you'll see in the next chapter, our addictions to self-image can sometimes lead us to abuse our sports to the point of self-destruction.

When we let our addictions control us, instead of the other way around, they can be a destructive force in our lives.

But in a lovely twist, we can trade an unhealthy addiction for a healthy one: our sports. Or, as our tire-changing friend Rebecca joked, "Some people work out because they can't handle a drug or alcohol addiction."

Our sports work beautifully as a alternative when they don't rob the other areas of our life in the bargain.

Sarah, a self-professed bike hound, says, "One of the things I've learned [from sports] is that we all deserve pursuits that make us happy and enrich our lives. I would not be where I am today without athletics. I'm not even sure I'd still be alive."

Sarah doesn't say that lightly. She comes from a family who modeled depression, alcoholism, and violent tempers. When she reached college, she was sure the path to transformation would be through substance abuse, so she dove right in. After about a year of bingeing on a buffet of alcohol and drugs, she was so unfit—mentally and physically—that she could hardly work the first two-hour shift of her new waitressing job. Fortunately, Sarah still had the presence of mind to pull an old Kmart bike out of the garage and start cycling every day; first five miles a day, gradually increasing to fifteen. But she was clear on one thing, and emphasized her point to her friends at every opportunity: she was *not* exercising. Not Sarah. No way. The bike was for stress relief, not fitness.

Fortunately, a rose is still a rose, no matter what you call that quintessential flower. The name is only nomenclature. Same with fitness, so I'm sure you can see where things are going here. A year or so later, Sarah realized that she enjoyed the cycling more than the drugs and drinking. Nice.

Not that I'm trying to make a moral point here about virtue, because as with most things in moderation . . . well, you can fill in the rest.

More than a decade has passed since then, and while Sarah still struggles with depression, a little sunshine on a couple of spinning wheels usually hits the spot.

Kicking a drug or alcohol addiction can make other challenges in life pale in comparison. Someone once told me that the first time they did heroin they thought, "This is my new best friend."

I'd prefer not to have a best friend like that, but I know that feeling from my sports, as does Joelle, the mountain climber and Harvard professor. She says this about her ascent of Tuckerman's Ravine: "An hour and a half in, I'm comfortably numb. It's the runners high—like an adrenalin spigot's been jammed 'on' internally. This must be what a 'fix' is to a drug addict. An old familiar friend, arms open wide."

If I have to choose my fix, I'd rather be hiking up Tuckerman's. The survival odds seem higher than heroin. And when you do—survive that is—Joelle says, "I've always found a direct correlation between extreme orientations and generalized achievement, perhaps the absence of risk aversion, perhaps the ability to sacrifice, perhaps, as the sociologist Durkheim would suggest: 'ability to defer gratification.'" Even better, it's an addiction that supports achievement in the long run.

Sign me up!

But sports can't always save us from addictions, not right away anyway.

 "Suddenly, this sweaty, happy, *alive* woman would appear in the house."

Molly, the founder of Girls on the Run, is all too familiar with addiction. As a child, Molly was jammed pretty tightly into what she's coined "the girl box." That's the place we squeeze ourselves into when we're trying to measure up to all those supposed assets a girl is meant to have—be thin, be blond and petite, be sexy, be demure, and so on. Her alcoholic mother offered no support. Then, when Molly was around fourteen, her mother started running. Suddenly, this sweaty, happy, *alive* woman would appear in the house. Soon enough her mother asked Molly to join her for a run. And that time with each other on the road became the grace in their day.

Yet running wasn't enough to let Molly out of the girl box.

As she says, "I took my first drink at age fifteen. Being drunk enabled me to feel comfortable in the girl box, so I did it for the next seventeen years. I never lost the running my mother had introduced me to, though. But there were times during workouts when I had the shakes from drinking too much the night before."

Molly "white-knuckled" her way through a Master's in Social Work, but then worked as a waitress instead, sleeping on a friend's couch.

"At thirty-two, I wanted to commit suicide."

After a particularly close brush with the idea of ending her life, she went for a run she's never forgotten. It was an oppressively hot Southern evening. Storm clouds were gathering in the sky. The leaves flipped upside down, exposing their pale underbellies.

 "For a *single* moment, as the weather closed in around her, Molly felt completely whole and content."

For a *single* moment, as the weather closed in around her, Molly felt completely whole and content. She burst into tears. And in that moment, she *knew* what she wanted to do. After beginning a twelve-step group, Molly began work on creating a curriculum-driven girl-empowerment program, with running at its core, where girls would have a safe space to come together and consider the choices in their lives. Her dream became reality. Molly let go of her addictions and found balance. She still runs, but often she does it with preteen girls. Not to mention with her own daughters.

Running couldn't prevent Molly's addictions, but it was there for her when she was ready to change direction, proving to be a better friend than alcohol. Running did not become her new addiction. Rather, the sport opened a window to Molly's own purpose in life: giving back.

SPREADING THE LOVE

On a frigid Saturday morning, I was wondering why I had signed up to be a "buddy" in the Girls on the Run 5k race. In the almost fifteen years since Molly started the nonprofit organization, Girls on the Run has grown into a national organization that has helped countless preteen girls develop their self-confidence and strength. Workshops on the pressing issues facing young girls, from peer pressure to body image, are wrapped around an end goal of training for a 5k race. On race day, the girls are each joined up with a volunteer (usually avid runners themselves, or at least avid believers in the possibilities of girls) who runs beside them, their own personal cheering section.

I have to admit, initially I didn't want to go. The run wasn't going to be a proper weekend workout, as I defined such a thing. The day was cold. I wanted to squeeze a quick intense run in and then stay home and read. But I'd signed up, so I went.

When I first met Jessie, the eleven-year-old girl I was running with, she ignored me in favor of hanging out with her friends. As I stomped my feet to keep warm, I wondered why I was even there.

"As I stomped my feet to keep warm, I wondered why I was even there."

Then the race started, and to my surprise, Jessie glued herself to my side, talking nonstop for the whole three miles. Among other things, I learned about her mother's nursing job, her new baby brother, her grandmother's dog, her dream of becoming a fashion designer, and that her favorite color was purple. As she talked, we ran a bit, walked a bit, up and back along the blowy East River in Manhattan. I was bundled up like the Michelin Man and having a great time. Jessie had never walked or run five kilometers in her whole life. But she never even considered giving up, and a little more than an hour after we started, we crossed the finish line together. Both of us were beaming. I ran home afterward, my legs stiff with cold.

The very best part of the deal was that I had a new window into running and what the pursuit meant to me. I felt lucky to be physically able to be a buddy. I felt privileged to have been present when Jessie crossed her first finish line.

I get so much from running, little had I known that I could get even more from it simply by sharing the gift with someone else. I had always wondered about people who were "pacers" in races. Why would they want to give up their race to do it for someone else, or some other group of people? Now I understand. Maybe I'll even look into it.

Like Molly, Mary Beth is another good example of giving back through her sports. Through her business, AlaVie Fitness, she gives women the opportunity to get healthy and build a community of like-minded women. But that's a business, so technically we might not call that giving *back*, even if her work benefits the women it serves. But Mary Beth goes further than that. Like me, on a recent Saturday morning she was wondering why she'd committed to develop a fundraising boot camp for the California Bay

Area Women's Sports Initiative (BAWSI—a great acronym if you say it out loud as if it were a word—a word that men sometimes like to use to describe women with opinions). BAWSI recruits college athletes to volunteer in less advantaged Bay Area neighborhoods, creating sports options for girls. They even developed a program for the girls' mothers, who were often sitting on the sidelines. They were thrilled to have their own reason to move around. The moment Mary Beth arrived at the event, she remembered why she'd given up her Saturday.

"There was so much passion, and what we are doing makes such a difference in people's lives," says Mary Beth. "This wouldn't happen if I were just pursuing money."

Indeed. Mary Beth inspires me to get cracking on giving back. And just as I'm having these thoughts, I discover that giving back might even be good for my health. How great is it when something we like turns out to be good for us as well? I'm all over the studies that show the salutary effects of chocolate, for example.

The scientific studies are piling up in which research has documented the positive effects that giving back, or volunteering, has on people's health. Altruism, it turns out, may be an important antidote to stress. Sharing our toys, as our parents taught us long ago, isn't just the right thing to do, it's the *healthy* thing to do.

For example, *The Journal of Health Psychology* published a study by Stanford University researchers at the Buck Center for

 "Sharing our toys, as our parents taught us long ago, isn't just the right thing to do, it's the *healthy* thing to do."

Research in Aging that found that community-service volunteering reduced mortality by as much as *60 percent*. A 2002 article in *Pain Management Nursing* reported the results of research showing that patients with chronic pain, when enlisted as peer volunteers to help other patients cope with their pain, experienced a reduction in pain, depression, and disability as a result. And in 2008, the journal *Psychosomatic Medicine* reported on research showing that HIV patients who volunteered to care for others and/or gave to charities experienced a slower disease progression.

Scientists call this phenomenon "the helper's high," an expression that comes from psychological research showing that "giving" actually produces endorphins (our old chemical friends from sports). Psychologist James Baraz, the cofounder of the Spirit Rock Meditation Center in Northern California, points out that compassion and caring about others does not, as we might expect, drain us; rather it fills us with energy. Why? Because, as Baraz says, "If you're not aligned with your values it eats at you. When you are [aligned], something in you grows and comes alive. Each one of us has our own hidden purpose inside and needs to uncover it and give it wings. Service is one of the things that gets us in touch with that most natural and true part of ourselves."

That last line has a certain resonance, doesn't it?

It certainly does with runner and human right's advocate Lisa Shannon. After seeing a story on *Oprah* about women brutalized by war in Africa's Congo, Lisa was inspired to turn her recreational running into something more. She founded Run for Congo Women, which has held races around the world to raise money to support Congolese women. Through Women for Women International, which is where the money goes, the women are taught essential life and work skills, from literacy and math to health education. Shannon was so drawn into the cause that now she volunteers full time, traveling often to the Congo to volunteer on the ground, in the communities in which these women live. Through her efforts, she is helping them build their independence and self-sufficiency. Her memoir, *A Thousand Sisters*, is also drawing international attention to their plight, helping spur political and social action.

Thich Nhat Hahn, a Buddhist teacher, activist, and author of many wonderful books, says, "Compassion is a verb." In other words, when we truly feel the suffering (and joy) of others, we are compelled to action.

Lisa's dedication is profound, but we don't all have to turn our lives completely around to give back.

For each one of us, the balance between giving back and taking care of ourselves is different. Giving is not a competition. In fact, it is a process by which we discover our values, and thus ourselves. At core, giving *is* about us; altruism is selfish, as the Dalai Lama has pointed out. Giving brings meaning into our lives, and meaning brings with it harmony and balance. A perpetual process of give and take, literally and metaphorically, physically and psychologically . . .

O n a trip to southern France, we woke up one morning to darkened skies. The normally deep blue water of the Côte d'Azure sea was a ferocious gray, peaked with foaming white caps. Trees bent before the wind's force, reminding me of what I strive for in yoga's tree pose. Rain *tock-tocked* on the wood porch outside our bedroom window.

We peered cautiously outside to assess the situation. The day did not look promising for a ride, which was disappointing since we'd flown our bikes all the way over and had hoped to ride every day. Then we thought of the coastal path. We had only walked short bits of it, never having the energy after our rides to spend any length of time exploring. At the front desk, we asked the hotel's concierge if he could arrange a taxi to take us to the beach town at the other end of the trail, about 10 kilometers away. When we told him we planned to run back to the hotel along the path, he seemed dubious.

The rain began to ease as the car took us to the start of our adventure, but the wind picked up. We set off with light hearts. The path climbed at first through a forest of Umbrella Pines, so-named because of their shape: short dark trunks and broad flat tops. The rain was more of a gentle mist, keeping us cool. After twenty minutes or so we burst out of the forest onto a path. Perched high above the sea, the path was rugged, narrow, and precipitous at times. Added to the tricky footwork required to stay upright was the wind, which threatened at any moment to lift us bodily into the air.

We bellowed back at the wind with delight as it embraced us, our feet firm on the earth even as we moved lightly around and over the obstacles. What a gift we had been given, the grace of those moments, the balance and harmony of being alone with the elements—ocean, sky and wind, the rocks and swaying trees. As if we were the first or last inhabitants of the world.

CHAPTER 5:

Fit Is the New Thin

"I see my body as an instrument, rather than an ornament."
—Alanis Morissette, musician

My bedroom floor is littered with discarded clothes and I'm standing sideways to the mirror, trying to determine whether the latest iteration of what I might wear tonight, a pair of black cords, make my just-got-my-period stomach look poochy, which will make my mind feel cranky. I looked great in these pants the day I tried them on, but now I can't get them off fast enough. I move to dresses. Oh yeah. Now we're talking.

Hello, legs. Did you have a nice workout this morning?

Yes, quite. And thanks for showing us off a little. After all, we've been carrying you around for quite a few hard miles.

Stomach, what stomach? I zip up a pair of these-boots-were-made-for-walking and head out to meet my friends.

BALANCE REDUX

We left balance in the last chapter, but as you no doubt can see, we're not quite finished with that issue. Our old frenemy body-image has yet to be introduced.

Just as we need balance in the structure of our lives, in how we commit to our sports and fit them into the rest of our lives, so do we also need to employ balance when we sit down to eat, put on our clothes, or look in the mirror. Because the unfortunate truth is that we're not always friends with how we feel about our appearance. Some days we just don't feel pretty, inside or out. Yet making an enemy of our body image does us no good. On a rational level I know that, yet I struggle at times to find peace and self-acceptance inside my skin. And when that happens, I sometimes enlist my sports almost as weapons against my negative self-image.

Exhibit A is a recent trip-and-fall knee injury I experienced that resulted in stitches and time off. It was my first spring run after the cross-country ski season. Before I left for that fateful run, I weighed myself. I had no real reason to beyond a generous dinner the evening before. My clothes all fit the same. I was just "checking." I weighed a few pounds more than the last time I'd "checked," and the news was immensely frustrating to me. Never mind that it was probably new muscle gained from a winter of cross-country skiing, or that I was still well within my healthy weight range. Instead, I got mad at myself. I set out on my run, my head clouded with negativity and self-criticism. And then what do you know, I tripped and fell, gashing my knee open to the bone and couldn't run for several weeks. Apparently, Karma patrol was in the neighborhood.

I felt badly about myself after one night of hearty eating and a winter of hard workouts, and yet I've felt beautiful in the middle of a delightfully indulgent and indolent vacation. Sometimes I forget the blindingly obvious, that beauty really *isn't* skin deep, quite the opposite. Just ask Molly, the founder of Girls on the Run who spent years battling her own way out of the tight confines of the "girl box." She puts it this way: "Beauty is an inside job." And she doesn't mean inside *that* box. She means inside our minds.

Beauty is really about balance.

"Why do only 12 percent of women think they look good in a swimsuit?"

We all know that beauty comes from within, from how we feel about ourselves, so why can't we remember that? Why do we have such a love-hate relationship with the way our bodies look? Why do only 12 percent of women think they look good in a swimsuit?

Ellis Cashmore, an expert in culture, media, and sport, puts the knotty image of body image this way in his book *Sport and Exercise Psychology: The Key Concepts*: "The way we perceive our own physical bodies is not a straightforward process, but rather like standing in a hall of mirrors: Our perceptions are reflections of how we believe others are perceiving and judging us. So physical self-perceptions are in many respects our perceptions of others' perceptions."

Our perceptions of others' perceptions—that's a brain twister to understand. So what we look like to ourselves is a function of how we think somebody else thinks we look. Somebody *else*, I might add, whose mind we are not inside and can never fully know.

Isn't that somewhere around at least two degrees of separation from reality? In any case, trying to sort out how we feel about our bodies can be worse than a hall of mirrors. Trying to measure up to a perception of another person's perceptions is a whole *not*-funhouse of distorted mirrors. The most likely outcome is self-delusion, and I don't mean of grandeur.

Body image delusion is so culturally ingrained that a recent study in the journal *Personality and Individual Differences* reported that even women whose psychological screenings raised no red flags for body image insecurity had MRI scans showing brain activity associated with the fear of getting fat, literally, when shown pictures of overweight women.

"Many women learn that bodily appearance and thinness constitute what's important about them, and their brain activity reflects that," said Diane Spangler, an author of the Brigham Young University study. "It's like the plant in my office," Spangler said. "It has the potential to grow in any direction, but actually only grows in the direction of the window—the direction that receives the most reinforcement."

We receive a barrage of constant reinforcement that we ought to be thin, thin, thin, and more thin still, and that changes the way we view ourselves.

The crux of the issue with body image is "perceived standards" of a thin ideal. Where on earth did these standards come from? Why haven't we figured out yet that a mass ideal could never be appropriate for all of us? And why is simply being fit not enough for too many of us?

LOST IN THE HALL OF MIRRORS

Where the ultra-thin standards come from seems both obvious and mysterious—our culture, our culture, our culture. But why? A fascinating question, no doubt, and one that has generated much brain power and ink in search of answers. Suffice to say, the thin ideal is deeply flawed.

Need proof? Hello, Barbie, you iconic every-girl's-fantasy doll. Did you know your plastic proportions, if applied to a regular woman, would result in a freakish being around seven feet tall, weighing a hundred pounds, with an eighteen-inch waist. Beautiful? Not!

The thin ideal is deeply flawed. A recent study showed that girls aged five to eight who played with a Barbie reported lower body-esteem and a greater desire to be thinner compared to girls of the same age who played with a doll that had more realistic body proportions. That does not bode well for the 90 percent of American girls who today own at least one Barbie, regardless of whether it's a Tennis Barbie or not; remarkable power for a small plastic toy, with sharp fingers and toes. And symbolic of a more deeply ingrained cultural bias that favors thinness over fitness.

We know the media, including many popular women's sports and fitness magazines, drive and feed the cultural obsession with thin. Yet for all our intellectual understanding, we can't stop obsessing. In the May 2008 issue of *Psychological Bulletin*, University of Wisconsin-Madison postdoctoral researcher Shelly Grabe and psychology professor Janet Hyde reported on their sweeping analysis of seventy-seven previous studies involving more than fifteen thousand subjects. In it, they found that exposure to media depicting ultra-thin actresses and models significantly increased women's concerns about their bodies, including how dissatisfied they felt and their likelihood of engaging in unhealthy eating behaviors, such as excessive dieting. Not only that, but they also found that the media has an even greater influence on women's body image today than it did in the 1990s.

 "'Women's displeasure with their bodies has become so common that it's now considered normal. . . .'"

We're "onto them," and still the media's power over how we internalize our feelings about our bodies is getting stronger.

"Women's displeasure with their bodies has become so common that it's now considered normal," says Grabe.

Truly, when I feel really good about myself physically, I'll sometimes think, *Am I deluding myself?* As if it's strange or weird to feel good about myself; to think when I look in the mirror, *Hey, nice legs.* When I don't feel good about myself, I'll believe that to get back to stasis I'll need to be hard on myself. This is obviously a delusional thought, but one that's hard to kick all the same. And as the studies show, I'm not alone in this issue.

The obsession with being thin can become so all-consuming for some women that their sports become more of a weapon they wield against themselves rather than a route to finding inner peace, with body image and so much else.

In *The Religion of Thinness*, author Michelle M. Lelwica looks at the slippery slide from good workout intentions into self-destructive behavior. This happens, she tells us, when "the primary aim [of the workout] is not peace of mind, body, and spirit, but thinness."

At the extreme, using our sports solely as a way to be thin can become a disease with a name: "exercise bulimia," a behavior in which a person exercises compulsively to purge the body of extra calories.

For Ruth Wallace the problem began in her teens, when she was a competitive tennis player. "Before college, I played tennis twice a day, waking up early to go before school, and then playing again in the evening," she says. "But *that* wasn't even enough. I also worked out for hours during the day—at lunch, when I had breaks between classes, or before or after tennis practices. I was determined to burn off every last calorie I'd eaten . . . and more, if I was lucky."

Exercise bulimia is considered a relatively "new" disease, and it's one that is typically hard to identify. After all, we've always been told that exercise is good for us, and doctors rarely ask us in detail about our exercise routines. Yet when the desire to exercise gets tangled up in a compulsive need to purge and an inability to tolerate periods of rest, then our sports are controlling us, not the other way around. And that's not a good thing. More and more doctors are recognizing exercise bulimia, and it is taking its place alongside anorexia and bulimia as a disease to watch for and treat.

Like Ruth, Julie Branch describes herself as a "serious athlete with a serious eating disorder." She has a hard time taking any days off because she won't let herself eat unless she's worked out—and not just worked out, but worked out to the point of exhaustion. So instead of taking rest or recovery days, Julie ends up with a few "starve-myself" days, which certainly isn't going to be any help when she works out the next day.

"No woman deserves to use her own commitment to exercise against herself," she says, and yet she knows that she does just that. Her relationship with her body has infected her relationship with her athletics. Instead of working out to feel strong and confident and good about her body, she exercises "to feel in control." Of what? "Of everything I can control," she says, "what I eat, how I look, how I feel physically." As if by being in control of those things, she will by some process of osmosis have more control over the rest of her life—work and relationships, for example. Yet she knows that's not true. She knows she'd be a better athlete and a healthier person, inside and out, if she ate more, slept adequately, and respected the concept of recovery days.

"The condition negatively affects my peace of mind, my relationship with others, and my athletic pursuits. This should be so unacceptable to me, that I should have unloaded the beast on my back a long time ago."

Julie is working hard on changing her attitude. Owning up to and talking about her challenge with others helps. And she's making good progress in learning to be at peace with her body. As in, she can take rest days and actually eat to keep her body fueled, even if it still feels uncomfortable. Baby steps.

Of course, Julie and Ruth are hardly alone in their struggles.

Exercise bulimia is just one manifestation of the depression that women are all too prone to suffer. Psychologists have pointed

"Psychologists have pointed out that women are two to three times as likely to suffer from depression as men."

out that women are two to three times as likely to suffer from depression as men. And one of the primary culprits is our excessive concern for social approval—which is intimately tied to a heightened concern with our physical appearance in general, and our weight in particular; which in turn fosters low self-esteem, which then can feed a woman's higher propensity toward depression; an ugly cycle that has perpetuated itself for several generations already, and shows no signs of letting up.

In 2009, the Women's Sports Foundation released a comprehensive report titled, *Her Life Depends on It II: Sport, Physical Activity, and the Health and Well-Being of American Girls and Women*, which delved deeply into the relationship between exercise and just about every facet of a woman's life, including depression. It turns out that exercise is a double-edged sword. All things being equal (in other words, balanced), women athletes, the report says, enjoy a greater sense of self-esteem and feel less depression than their sedentary peers.

As athletes we know this to be true. We feel good about ourselves as a result of our sports. As we saw in chapter 2, this good feeling is even scientifically quantifiable. Yet if we are honest with ourselves, that good feeling is a matter of equilibrium, and when things get out of whack, we can upset the equation. Athletes, for example, are also at greater risk of eating disorders, the report points out. And eating disorders are often the handmaidens of depression in women. In fact, excessive exercise can be a red flag for depression, low self-esteem, and poor body image. As the report says, "In essence, sports participation in moderation enhances mental health; in excess, it may (literally) be overkill."

In *Woman: An Intimate Geography*, Natalie Angier offers up an interesting perspective on women's depression in general.

"Aggression and depression sound like two different, even polarized phenomena, but they're not. Depression is aggression turned inward, directed against the self, or the imagined, threatening self." Angier explores and debunks many of the theories of the higher male propensity toward aggression, arguing that social conditioning may have just as much to do with women's seeming passivity. Women's depression may be our natural, but socially unacceptable, aggression turned inward. And when we hate our own bodies enough to damage them physically by depriving them of food, or exercising excessively, that's nothing but an aggression against our selves.

Eating disorders, using our sports against ourselves, how depressing, literally. We need to find the emergency exit from that hall of mirrors, but like all funhouses, what looks like the way out is often just another blind alley reflected to infinity. In plain speak, those we assume have our best interests in mind may not actually be directing us to the nearest exit.

IF YOU JUST LOST A LITTLE WEIGHT . . .

When I was a little girl, I wanted to be a ballerina. After all, ballerinas were the epitome of beauty, or so I thought—tall (I had no idea that was the optical illusion of being on point), thin and delicate (as much as I loved the vigor of summer camp, it felt almost too robust for how girls ought to be), and that perfect chignon hair (so unlike my own harem-scarem curls, which refused to succumb to direction). Despite my pleading, my parents would not allow me to take ballet classes. I tried showing them how serious I was by practicing the different positions out of a book I laid open on my bedroom floor in front of me. All to no avail. I suspected they thought I wasn't tall, thin, or delicate enough. Or maybe it was my hair. For years, I stewed about my missed opportunity to be a *prima*.

Then, as an adult, I had a brief fling with the tutu. And I can tell you, it was not pretty—and it had nothing to do with my looks. I took a few ballet classes with a friend of mine, and frankly I was appalling. For one thing, despite my diligent yoga practice, my hamstrings were so tight from running that once my foot was up on the bar, the notion that I could bend my torso gracefully over my leg, nose to knee, was completely out of the question. And that was just a warm-up stretch. We hadn't even gotten to the "real ballet" yet, the *grand jeté,* the *grand battement.* It quickly became clear that I was not going to be gracefully, or otherwise, lifting one leg above my ear anytime soon.

When I mentioned to my father that I was taking ballet classes, he said, "Oh, your mother never wanted you to take ballet as a child. She didn't want to subject you to the ballet mistresses always telling everyone to be skinnier. She'd had enough of that when she took ballet as a girl."

Say what? I'd never known that my parents had a reason for not letting me take the classes, let alone a *good* one. I was quite thin as a girl, even if I didn't think so at the time. I shudder to think how I would have reacted to being told to lose weight.

And my parents weren't wrong. A recent study by the Medical College of Wisconsin showed that 32 percent of professional ballet dancers suffer severe disordered eating and 18 percent reported going long periods without, well, periods. Not having a period sounds pretty great at first blush, a nice hassle-reduction, but really an irregular menstrual cycle is a sign of excessive thinness and malnourishment; and amenorrhea, as losing your period is called, is one of the three hallmarks (along with disordered eating and premature bone loss) of a growing health syndrome called the Female Athlete Triad, a.k.a. FAT, and a more apt acronym could never be.

Ballet is hardly the only culprit. Lots of other sports, especially the so-called "appearance" sports, like running, gymnastics, and figure skating, for example, are guilty of cultivating the FAT. Needless to say, the women who fall prey to the triad do not fare well, either mentally or physically. This is not the place for the harrowing examples of FAT gone wild, suffice to say that it can result in a succession of debilitating injuries as estrogen plummets and bone density diminishes; and, in the worst cases, FAT is fatal.

But as I said in the beginning, this is a book about ordinary woman, and in our ordinary ways, many of us have struggled with the less severe manifestations of the FAT. Because not only is the media projecting images that squirrel their way into our psyche, internal voices telling us how we ought to look, creating unrealistic, even preposterous standards, too often there are *actual* voices outside our head telling us we just aren't thin enough.

First stop: coaches.

Rebecca, the world champion adventure racer, had a college running coach who once said to her, "You ate two whole pieces of pizza?!" He wasn't asking, he was *accusing*. He then proceeded

"'You ate two whole pieces of pizza?!' He wasn't asking, he was *accusing*."

to tell all the women on his running team that they were "fat and slow." Just a guess, but I'm thinking that he was not a coach who stayed up late composing his motivational talks.

Rebecca quit the running team and went through, as she puts it, "a bit of an eating disorder" period. To this day, this hyper-fit woman will get her new race kit and wonder, "Does my race kit make me look fat?" Impossible, unless we're going to start calling Jennifer Aniston fat, too.

Of course, Rebecca's coach is hardly the only sterling example of such nurturing behavior toward his women athletes. Robin Campbell, a former Wall Street broker, is a five-foot-eight, 116-pound speedster. She's basically a beautiful string bean with muscles, and has been all her life.

"Our college running coach was always telling us we needed to lose weight," Robin says.

College was twenty years ago for her, but his voice is lodged way too deeply for a mere couple of decades to mute it. I can hear her channeling his voice when she says to me, "Ugh, I'm fat. I gained four pounds when I couldn't run because of my stress fracture." Mind you, she was still biking like mad at her gym. And some might even say the extra few pounds were a welcome addition. But it will be a few years yet before she thinks so. We can take a moment to thank her coach for helping out on that front.

What are these coaches smoking? We look at other women, whether friends or strangers, and we shake our heads and think, "That's just crazy! You look great." And we can clearly see what our friends can't—that they should be happy with their bodies. Yet, how often do we let these negative messages infect our own self-image, even to a small degree? Guilty as charged.

""I can remember being in the second grade and my aunts lining me and my two cousins up and telling us who was thinnest."

Unfortunately, it's not just coaches and ballet mistresses who can get inside our heads. How about family?

Texas Rebecca, who faced her fear of changing tires, once weighed over 250 pounds. As a child and teenager she struggled with being heavy. "I can remember being in the second grade and my aunts lining me and my two cousins up and telling us who was thinnest. Another time I was changing clothes and my cousin, who had lost weight, decided to try on my pants. They were huge on her. She walked out in front of all my aunts and I heard them all burst into loud laughter."

And how about even closer to home—mothers, anyone?

When Sandra Monaghan, a downhill skier and professional cellist, got her first waitressing job at fourteen, her mother said, "The uniform is perfect for you. The black on the bottom will make your hips and bum look smaller, and the white top will compensate for your flat chest."

That's what a friend of mine calls a "depth charge"—that is, something that *almost* sounds like a compliment, but in actuality carries with it a powerful explosive designed to be a direct hit on your self-confidence.

Thirty years later, even though Sandra is tall and lithe (at five-foot-seven and 117 pounds), she still hears her mother's voice in her head every time she puts on a pair of pants (mostly black, of course), and pulls up the straps of her 32A bra. If Sandra's size-4 bum is big, then I'll eat my ski hat.

Mothers' voices have a special place inside our head, but friends, spouses, lovers, and really anyone we respect and trust, anyone whose opinion matters deeply to us, can have a deleterious impact on our self-image.

For Mary Reese, a teacher and volleyball coach (who no doubt is more supportive than other coaches we've met here) had her own self-image naysayer in the form of a high school boyfriend. A wrestler with his own eating disorder (sadly common because of stringent weight restrictions), her boyfriend was "recovering" from a downward weight spiral when Mary met him. Theoretically, says Mary, he was committed to being healthy. Instead, he channeled everything into obsessive fitness, including Mary, who already participated in everything from running to volleyball.

"I could never work out enough to meet his high standards," she says. "But I was star-struck, so I believed everything he said. He made me feel like I wasn't skinny enough or toned enough. I can't tell you how many times I cried myself to sleep, wanting nothing more than to please him, just once."

Fortunately for Mary, they broke up five years later. At first she was heartbroken, then she realized how much happier she was, not to mention how much fitter. "Working out became fun again," says Mary. "And," she adds, "so did dating!"

Then there's Kristy's equally "nurturing" former boyfriend. When she was in college, he told her, "If you gain ten pounds, I'll drop you like a bad habit." Thankfully, she dropped *him* like a bad habit instead, and today she's a member of the U.S. Women's National Bandy Team (not to mention inspiring little girls to be hockey players). "I still struggle with self-image issues," she says, "but I feel best when I feel 'fit.'"

Raise your hand if, like me, you're also worn out on the media-generated angst, insidious ballet instructors, trash-talking coaches, and depth-charging loved-ones. Fitness fits in our lives for so many great reasons; why tarnish our relationship with sports by using it against ourselves. How, then, do we stop? I'm sensing a familiar presence . . .

Balance, my old friend, thanks for stopping by.

FINDING OUR "JUST RIGHT"

I thought of Rebecca's not-motivational coach the other night when I was wolfing down pizza, feeling like I couldn't get enough to restoke after putting in a fifty-mile running week. I froze for a moment during my dinner. *Hmmm?* I was feeling great, like I was in excellent shape and looked good, strong and healthy.

But maybe . . . I was . . . *deluded?*

Clunk.

That was the sound of me dropping off the cliff of confidence, accidentally blaring Radio KFKD. *Maybe I shouldn't eat the pizza at all. I don't need that much food. I'll get fat. Or maybe I can just have one piece, even though I'm still awfully hungry, and the cheese and veggies and homemade crust with the crunchy polenta dusted on top tastes so delicious.*

I fought this little internal battle with myself for a few minutes, my pizza cooling on the plate, until I switched stations to Radio K-GrrrT. *Just stop all this nonsense! Eat your pizza! All this running and you still can't relax into your dinner?—don't be silly. Enjoy it,*

> "She had fun, just fun, no dialogue in her head about not being good enough or thin enough, no counting how many calories she burned."

for goodness sake. Well the voice might have used stronger language than that last, given that it was in my head. But you get the point.

Because guess what, we *need* food. Food is our friend. And if we're working out hard, we need to replenish. As strong, balanced athletes, we're trying to avoid getting FAT, not necessarily *fat.*

Remember Ruth, the tennis player we met at the beginning of the chapter who suffered from exercise bulimia? Her strained relationship with sports and eating was interrupted when she went to college. There was no tennis team, and she was simply too busy with schoolwork to pursue sport recreationally, let alone obsess over calories. She focused her attention elsewhere, and the hiatus did her good. When she returned to sports after college, she had a healthy new mind-set and healthier eating habits. At twenty-nine, she borrowed a friend's bike and went for a short ride. She had fun, just fun, no dialogue in her head about not being good enough or thin enough, no counting how many calories she burned.

She loved it so much, she returned the friend's bike and bought her own, a Kmart Huffy bike. "I signed up for the thirty-five-mile Five Boro Bike Tour in New York City," says Ruth. "A bit ambitious, I know, but I didn't even really know what thirty-five miles meant. I rode the whole tour alone. One of my tires got a flat, but I just kept on riding. I was hooked. It was all just so amazing, being outside, seeing the city, feeling my legs working on the bike."

The Huffy went back to Kmart (that's quite a return policy), she bought a better bike, and developed a new appreciation for food. Then came triathlons, then marathons. She now finds solace, strength, and confidence in training. "Instead of demonizing food, I understand that it's the fuel that enables me to participate in the sports I love."

Indeed, because even if you are trying to lose weight to improve your performance for a particular race, thinner is not always better. Exercise physiologists generally agree that for sports in which less weight can improve performance, like running, cycling, cross-country skiing, or swimming, weight loss can increase speed, but only up to a certain point. Too thin means your body is literally feeding on itself to find energy, and not on the food you're eating, since you're not eating enough. In other words, we're losing strength, rather than gaining it. The equation is simple, but one that we may overlook through inattention, or on purpose, because we're caught up in wanting to lose weight. The equation is called "energy availability," which is defined as energy intake (yes, that means through food) minus energy expended (via exercise, oh yes, and via living and breathing and digesting and walking around and working). And yes, the energy availability equation is really just another cut at balance. For nonelite athletes, flirting with excessive thinness can start to look suspiciously like obsession.

Karen Fleet, a lawyer in her early fifties, is a prime example. After her third child was born, she weighed two hundred pounds and was unhappy with how she looked and felt. She took stock of herself. "I thought, I can resign myself to decrepitude or I can own my body again."

She started running ten miles a day, no days off; and swimming one mile a day, no days off. Yes, I do mean running ten miles *and* swimming one mile, every day, no days off. Now this might be a respectable training load for a competitive world-class athlete, but maybe not such a great idea for the rest of us, even if we're in good shape to start with. In Karen's case, she went from zero to sixty overnight. She lost, as she says, "a gazillion" pounds and "felt ridiculously proud," even though she was stick thin. Her friends thought she looked terrible. To add injury to insult—literally—she ended up with a stress fracture as a result of the demands she was putting on her body. The injury was a red flag, letting Karen know that she had lost balance in her life, and she was forced to rethink her workout and weight loss stratagems. In fact, she changed her whole approach to running. Instead of using running to control her weight, the quiet time alone on the road became an opportunity for healthy self-reflection.

"It's through sports that I realize how blocked I am in different areas of my life," says Karen. "Suddenly I think, 'Wow, you grossly underestimated what you are capable of doing.' The breakthroughs, where I have to reassess what I'm capable of, have happened in sports."

And with that change in perspective, Karen is eating better and running moderate distances four to six times a week. When she finally built up in a measured way to running her first marathon, she was ecstatic. "It took me a lot of years to get to that finish line. And I definitely got there when I was in the right place."

She'd found her "just right" place, or middle path. Just like a rose, balance by any other name is just as balanced. Nope, I never said I was a poet.

Here's another middle path. Christine Jeremie, a former investment banker and runner, took up running at age thirty-eight because she didn't want to get fat as she got older. Until then she had never done any sports. She burst onto the New York running scene with a bang, doing a 3:13 for her first marathon. Now she places in any race she competes in. "Why do anything halfway, even if it's just taking out the trash," is Christine's philosophy. Her goals in running moved almost immediately beyond fat-prevention, which she hardly thinks about anymore, and into the nuanced balance between training enough to improve her speed, and not so much that she gets slower.

The balanced place is different for each of us. That's the essence of being individuals, after all. Our individual bodies have a way of letting us know what's too much. Karen has maintained her equilibrium for more than fifteen years now and her weight, at a healthy 135 pounds, is just right for her.

Kelly, the coach and professional athlete, doesn't even own a scale. "It can make us too obsessive to be on that thing every day," she says.

We know that feeling good about ourselves has less to do with the numbers on the scale than whether or not it's one of those "just right" days or a "just wrong" day. Some days, a seemingly small thing can shift our focus in an instant.

Allison Pattillo actually felt the shift from negative body image to positive after a single phone call. She'd just come home feeling bloated after a Southern Thanksgiving feast. A freelance writer, she was waiting to hear about whether a possible column she'd submitted had been accepted. Nothing. Empty inbox. Too disheartened to contemplate doing anything else, she let lethargy take hold.

"I didn't want to go for a run," says Allison, "I decided I was just going to sit around, eat bonbons, and be fat instead. Then I get a phone call from the *Army Times* saying they wanted to run my column. I immediately went for a celebratory run, held my head high, and felt thinner and stronger. Completely whacked, but true."

Lisa, of the Spinster Chronicles, manifests her body image lethargy in a different way.

> "'I slip into a pair of sleek and defined hamstrings the way Sarah Jessica Parker slips into the latest piece of haute couture.'"

"Sometimes, when I haven't been working out for a long stretch of time and I'm not feeling good about my body, I find myself fixated on material things. I notice a woman's jewelry and develop a craving for diamond studs. But training changes all of that. I slip into a pair of sleek and defined hamstrings the way Sarah Jessica Parker slips into the latest piece of haute couture."

Our moods have more to do with how we feel about our bodies than the actual condition of our bodies. We find our equilibrium when we consciously work to accept who we are, inside and out. When we forget that we are working out to be strong and peaceful, things can go awry. When our sports are about controlling how we look from the outside in, starving ourselves of food, we also starve ourselves of pleasure. We turn our sports into weapons, deployed against the enemy of our weight. We lose sight of the joy to be found in our sports, not to mention in food. We forget that really it's what is inside of us that controls how we feel.

"A" IS FOR ATHLETIC

We think we want to be picture perfect, but when we really think about it, what does that mean? Is perfect all dolled up in our Sex and the City wear? Or is it a pair of defined hamstrings.

When I climb, I get bruises—big black-and-blue, egg-shaped bumps on my shins and knees and elbows. My knuckles get scraped up, and my nails look torn and frazzled. I remember finishing the West Coast Trail, a gorgeous hike in Pacific Rim National Park in British Columbia, and being thrilled about the prospect of shaving my legs for the first time in a week, only to discover that underneath the perma-layer of mud I'd been carrying around, there were all sorts of bug bites and cuts and purpled welts hiding out. I won't even get into the condition of my feet when I'm running a lot. I always feel like I need to tip the long-suffering pedicurist extra for putting up with them.

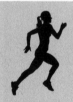

"I'd rather risk the covert stares from strangers wondering at my somewhat battered condition than sacrifice the joy of feeling my body in motion."

Sometimes I'm embarrassed by the way my sports "mark" me, but then I remember the stories behind those temporary imperfections—the viney roots I've tumbled over and the stinging nettles I've brushed through, the scaly rock walls I've cozied up against and the chain rings that have bitten into my calves in a sudden stop—and I don't care. I'd rather risk the covert stares from strangers wondering at my somewhat battered condition than sacrifice the joy of feeling my body in motion.

Our sports should be our friends, and like our friends, they are a form of spiritual and physical nourishment, one that empowers us to see our beauty, inside and out, no matter whether we fit some made-up ideal.

Laural, the adventure mentor, spent her high school years envying women with larger breasts. She even developed some animosity toward bra companies, which seem to think that small-breasted women don't deserve much in the pretty or sexy department—unless, of course, it comes in the padded or push-up style. After all, isn't there something wrong with us if we don't want to be bigger?

"Years of schooling trained me to look down at papers returned to my desk and feel good when I saw an A. But if you're a girl looking down at your chest, and *not* at your desk, that "A" does not elicit the same joy."

Being athletic changed Laural's mind on the issue.

"Sure, I see women in the locker room with breasts I might trade mine in for, but now it's more of an idle thought, like admiring a woman with a great haircut. I am fine in the breasts I happened into. Lately I am thinking that "A" is for Athletic. It's not that my breasts are doing calisthenics on their own, but that I share a breast size with some pretty fit Olympic athletes."

When we are comfortable in our skin, we are no longer obsessed with comparing ourselves to others, for worse and for better.

As Donna, the avid climber says, "When running up a hill, I love the look of my leg muscles working."

How much better is being strong and healthy than cultivating an emaciated frailty?

The Women's Sports Foundation study I mentioned earlier found that the more time girls spend participating in team sports, the higher their self-esteem. And a 2008 University of Florida study found that the simple act of exercise, and not the level of fitness itself, can convince us that we look better. In fact, even if we don't achieve workout milestones such as losing fat, gaining strength, or boosting cardiovascular fitness, we are likely to feel just as good about our bodies as a more athletic woman. As Heather Hausenblas, the exercise psychologist who conducted the study, said, "You would think that if you become more fit that you would experience greater improvements in terms of body image, but that's not what we found. It may be that the requirements to receive the psychological benefits of exercise, including those relating to body image, differ substantially from the physical benefits."

And that's not all. According to a 2009 University of Pennsylvania School of Medicine study, breast cancer survivors who lift weights regularly feel better about their bodies and their appearance and are more satisfied with their intimate relationships. Not only that, the survivors' better body image was unrelated to how much muscle strength they actually built.

"The results suggest that the act of spending time with your body was the thing that was important—not the physical results of strength," said senior author Kathryn Schmitz.

One more, because three's a charm and the data's compelling—a 2007 study by researchers at University of Ohio and East Carolina University looked at college women who suffered from social physique anxiety—a disorder in which someone chronically worries that others are critiquing his or her body. The research suggested that this group of women were more likely to attend and stick with an exercise class where the instructor emphasized the health benefits of the workout (as in, this will make you fit), over improved appearance (as in, this will tighten your butt), even if those women chose the class in hopes of improving their physique.

The "why" of why we engage in our athletics matters.

As Colleen Grazioso, a runner and former Wall Street banker says, "I want to look good. Fit. Healthy. Not necessarily thin. I derive self-confidence from being in control of how I look—not from being thin."

 "To be a certain weight is so much less important than plain old confidence, from which beauty really flows."

Internalizing that knowledge, particularly with respect to our weight, is a challenge for many of us. To be a certain weight is so much less important than plain old confidence, from which beauty really flows. And, guess what?—Sports give us that confidence.

Geeta Ling, a senior executive for a curriculum development company, took up running in college because of body image issues, hoping that running would keep her thin. Then something strange and wonderful happened. Being out on the road became something more than a means to control her weight. She did her first half-marathon and discovered a whole new piece of running. The race ignited her competitive spirit, and suddenly running wasn't about looking good anymore, it was about so much more. It was about feeling stronger and healthier. It was about thinking, "I can do something that other people can't do."

"It is something for *myself*, a solitary thing, a way to escape, to de-stress, to meditate," she says. Now in her late thirties, Geeta has moved far beyond her initial purpose for lacing up her shoes. "Running," she adds, "is when I have epiphany moments."

BYE, BYE, BARBIE

During the *Vogue*-thin Twiggy days of the 1960s, Rebecca Bailey, an emergency room mental health counselor in her late forties, says she didn't really have the option to model this frail ideal, not that she wanted to. As a matter of fact, Rebecca says she liked being muscular and fit. It was what earned her an athletic scholarship to college in discus throwing, which is a sport for big strong girls. Even as a teen and young adult, Rebecca had the self-confidence to realize that Twiggy was not a healthy role model. Today, the mother of three is a role model herself, but for what she calls "larger-size bodies." Not only does she compete in triathlons, she now also teaches a class called "Triathlon 101." Her message? "If I can do it, so can you."

And since we're thinking about one Rebecca, let's circle back to our courageous tire-changing Rebecca, who we last saw being shamed by her cousins and aunts. What, she wondered, could she do about her weight? Exercise? Unlikely, she thought. Rebecca assumed running was impossible for her to do because she only saw size-4 girls jogging at the local park. But once she mustered the courage to don running shoes, she realized that the sport wasn't about size. Running was about stamina. And she had that. After that, running like a girl stopped being about running like a *size-4* girl. While she's still not a small woman by today's "perceived standards," she says she derives a certain pleasure out of passing a Barbie-thin woman when she's out for a run.

Fit is the new thin. Fit is the new black. *Fit* is the point.

> **"Refreshingly, the media, which has traditionally not been our friend in reinforcing the beauty of different body types, has started to take notice of so-called 'real women.'"**

Refreshingly, the media, which has traditionally not been our friend in reinforcing the beauty of different body types, has started to take notice of so-called "real women." I might even go so far as to say that we are becoming an "in" thing. Dove soap, for example, initiated its "self-esteem movement" to educate and encourage women to develop a positive relationship with their beauty. To show its commitment, Dove advertisements feature "real women," a far more varietal array of faces than are usually found on billboards.

And if more companies don't begin to follow in Dove's footsteps, legislation may force the change. In March 2010, the Healthy Media for Youth Act, a piece of bipartisan legislation, was introduced in Washington, D.C., to establish a national task force that would develop voluntary guidelines to promote healthier media images for girls and women. True, "voluntary" doesn't sound quite as strong as we'd like, but it's a start. The legislation, which was developed in collaboration with the Girl Scouts, is a part of the Scouts' wider effort known as Live Healthy, Lead Healthy. Launched at the federal, state, and local levels, its aim is to engage politicians and communities around key health and well-being issues affecting girls.

Even in France, where women supposedly don't get fat, politicians tried to outlaw the promotion of extreme thinness in 2006, causing great hue and cry from the fashion industry. While the legislation, which was to apply to fashion magazines, advertisers, and websites that were found guilty of "inciting others to deprive themselves of food to an excessive degree," did not pass, the fact that the effort was made speaks volumes. In 2005, Spain banned too-thin women from the catwalk. And Italy, too, has tried its hand at campaigns to encourage a healthier media image of women.

Personally, I welcome all efforts, because this is an issue I still struggle with too, as if you hadn't already guessed. That's me, subtle like a sledgehammer, as one of my friends is prone to say. When the frustrations and anxieties pile up, and I'm looking for someone or something to blame, what do you know; it must be that I'm fat.

Actually, there was a time I used to buy my clothes a size too big because I was convinced that tomorrow I would be an out-of-shape Pillsbury dough-girl. My pants would gape open around the back of my waist when I sat down. My skirts would whirl in circles when I walked anywhere, ending up askew. I thought I was being smart. Saving money on clothes that I was going to outgrow any day.

 "Food and I have become much better friends. So have my body and me."

Not anymore. *Phew.* I buy clothes that fit me *now,* as in, *to-day.* My workouts are not about burning calories; they're my own version of hedonism, joyful and rejuvenating. Food and I have become much better friends. So have my body and me. After all, I've only got the one body, I can be unhappy with it, or I can be happy with it. The choice is up to me. I choose the latter. Okay, I choose the latter the majority of the time, say 80 percent. The other 20 percent of the time is backsliding, but hey, that gives me something to work toward, right?

When we look inward for our value, instead of outward, we discover the gorgeous freedom of the exercise-and-a-balanced-diet approach to life. And when we aren't afraid of our own strong muscles, or indeed any way that our body might look, then we accept control over our lives and how we appear in the world. After all, we come in an amazing and wonderful array of shapes and sizes.

Sitting in the shadow of Istanbul's history-steeped Blue Mosque, its dome bruise-colored in the sunset light, the ancient *hamam* breathes quiet antiquity from its impenetrable stone walls. Inside this cavernous Turkish bath, the twenty-first century is a future yet to come. After changing into nothing more than a towel and a pair of slip-on sandals, I emerge from the locker room. Wrapped modestly in my towel, I join the varietous bustle of women who flow in and out of the double doors, releasing a cloudy puff of steam each time the doors swing open.

Inside, the air is thick and humid. Soft light from somewhere high above catches droplets of steam in its beams. The room is enormous, tiled floor to ceiling in gray-veined marble. Its vaulted ceiling soars over an enormous marble slab platform, on which thirty or so women recline, some alone, eyes closed; others chatting, their voices echoing and muffled at the same time. A murmured blend of languages I recognize, even if I can't understand them, and others I can't identify. Around the edges of the platform lie about a dozen women who are being scrubbed by other women, foam bubbling up around them.

Everyone is naked, or might as well be. The scrubbers wear assorted styles of cotton underwear, from string bikini to high-waisted grandma, but the underwear is soaked through with steam and sweat and water, and hangs from their bums, loose and transparent. The women being scrubbed wear nothing but soap bubbles. Their towels lay off to the side, lumpy and damp.

I grew up going to the local pool, where my mother and I showered in communal showers, but still, I have never seen such a cornucopia of naked women in one place. Not just that, but all the women project an ease with their bodies, a sense of perfect comfort, lying naked among strangers. Instead of feeling vulnerable and exposed, as I assumed I would with all my flaws on display, the soft gray room creates an immediate aura of ease. Worse than my own discomfort, I thought I might feel critical of the other women, the way I sometimes am, as if in finding fault with others I can salve my own insecurities. Instead, I feel beautiful here in this Turkish bath, with so many women comfortable inside their skins, and therefore gorgeous. A gentle reminder of the thousand-and-one ways of lovely.

CHAPTER 6:

Chicking the Boys

*"Bicycling has done more to emancipate women than
any one thing in the world . . . A woman awheel is the
picture of untrammeled womanhood.*
—Susan B. Anthony, suffragist, 1896

For three days straight, we'd been making the climb up Mount Kilimanjaro, going *"poli-poli,"* Swahili for "slowly," to acclimatize to the altitude. Of the twelve people who had started this guided hike up Africa's highest mountain, my former husband and I were two of only four climbers remaining who planned to complete the final ascent to the peak—nearly 20,000 feet above sea level. The thought alone sent a buzz through my system.

The alarm bleeped at 3:00 AM and I was instantly wide awake, nerves jangling with anticipation. I had been lucky with the altitude. Not so "D," my ex, who woke with a massive headache—a hallmark of altitude sickness. The morning was dark and cold, and we were bundled in every layer we'd brought, only our eyes visible. The trail climbed in steep switchbacks over black lava rock and rubble, which shifted beneath our feet as we walked, increasing the effort required. Now our slow speed was enforced by the altitude and terrain. After about an hour, D stopped, pulled down his scarf, and dry retched at the side of the trail.

"I'm done," he said, "this is as far as I go." His voice sounded wobbly.

The guide had told us this could happen to any one of us, but we'd be fine once we retreated to a lower altitude. There was nothing I could do to make him feel better, at least not physically.

I thought, *What is he trying to say to me? Does he expect me to turn back with him?* Our guide was waiting for our decision. Physically, I felt fine. After so much painstaking planning and effort, I wanted so much to reach the top. Was I a terrible wife for wanting to finish what we had come to do together? Would he feel abandoned? Resentful? Was it my duty to stay back?

I reasoned to myself that if our positions were reversed, it would be different. He would no doubt continue on. And I would encourage him to. We *expect* men to accomplish things. To overcome hardship and challenge, to finish at all costs. But I wasn't a man. I was a woman, and that came with its own set of expectations: be a good wife, nurturing, self-sacrificing, protector of the male ego. What would the consequences be if I "bettered" him, if I soldiered on like he would have?

I hesitated, deferring to him, waiting for him to decide on my behalf; but he just kept looking at me, inscrutable in the dark.

"I'll come back down with you," I said. I wanted to cry.

As soon as we reached the lower hut, he felt restored to health, and we continued down the mountain at a brisk clip, conquering in one day what had taken us three days of hard hiking to cover. He felt rejuvenated, and I defeated—resentful even.

He didn't ask me to retreat. And we never spoke of it.

I had caved under the weight of hundreds of years of deep cultural conditioning all by myself. Small comfort to know that I am hardly the first or last woman to hold herself back in the service of a man's ego.

When it comes to sports (never mind everything else), the dynamic between the sexes can be complicated, to say the least. Sometimes the relationship between us women and the men in our lives is as smooth and easy as a companionable game of Frisbee on a summer afternoon. At other times, it can be so fraught that it forces a wedge between otherwise happy couples. At their worst, gender dynamics in sports can be a blatant example of sexism, even downright misogyny.

Why *are* sports a particular friction point? And why do we sometimes allow men's voices to interfere with the pursuit of our athletics? The reasons are many, and all owe quite a bit to the too-long-entrenched stereotypes of the masculine and feminine ideal. One thing is sure, by holding ourselves back from reaching the top

"At their worst, gender dynamics in sports can be a blatant example of sexism, even downright misogyny."

of the proverbial mountain, we perpetuate outdated gender roles and expectations that no longer have relevance—in *or* outside of sports.

WE *WILL* VELOCIPEDE

Why *do* we hold back? Well, often it's because as women we are more likely to define ourselves through our relationships, through the roles we fill in conjunction with men. Studies have actually shown that we tend to see ourselves as girlfriends, wives, and mothers first. Whether we're conscious of it or not, we may hold ourselves back in sports, unwilling to perform at our best, because our best might threaten the men in our lives and upset the balance of power in the relationship. Defining ourselves as *partners* to our men is not inherently bad, we simply need to be sure we don't let that definition work against our own interests—in sports as in all realms of our lives where we might hesitate in exerting our true capacity.

Competition among women exists, of course. What makes the male-female dynamic different is the insidious sexism of gender stereotypes, a programming so subtle we are often not aware of all the ways we are perpetuating the gender dichotomy—remember Barbie's effect on women's self-esteem? And Molly Barker's girl box?

Numerous studies have shown that the competitive drive of men from the Western world is higher than that of women. Notice I said "Western," because here's the rub. A recent study that isolated for the social conditioning of our patriarchal society looked at the competitive drives of men and women in a patriarchal society versus that of a matriarchal society (in which the leadership roles are taken by women). The results were revealing—competitive drive ended up being a function of the gender bias in the society.

"The results were revealing—competitive drive ended up being a function of the gender bias in the society. "

In patriarchal systems, where not only leadership but lineage is the province of men, they were—surprise, surprise—more competitive. In matrilineal culture, the opposite held true: women were more competitive. So competitiveness may not be about X or Y (a little chromosomal humor). Sadly, the study also found that true matriarchal societies no longer exist.

This is not to say there aren't significant differences between men and women. How we approach a competitive challenge, for one, may be different. For example, some research suggests that women are biologically predisposed to be more risk averse than men. When men are faced with a challenge (class 6 rapids, say), their bodies will typically produce adrenaline, that torqued-up "fight or flight" chemical that causes them to mimic banshees, hooting and hollering and running around in a show of frenetic excitement—no offense to banshees. But, and here's the *but*, when women are confronted by the same kind of challenge, our bodies produce acetylcholine, a totally different kind of chemical, which makes us want to throw up instead. Nice. And apparently, the urge to throw up helps us take time to mull over decisions instead of leap into the unknown, whooping it up as we go. Of course, we all know testosterone plays a role as well, and we'll get to that.

So maybe some of what looks like competitiveness in men is really just a lot of sound and fury, while us women are quietly toting up the cost-benefits of the challenge on our mental abacus, waiting to jump into the fray when the time is right. Watch out for us!

Not to blind you with science, but here is one more illuminating bit of information on the gender-stereotyping front, this from a study by a father-daughter team of researchers out of the University of Miami: not only men, but also women, support the established gender hierarchy in our society. And no matter the gender, the more entrenched a person is in the current social hierarchy, the more hostile they are to women who violate sex-role expectations. The study goes on to make a distinction between "benevolent sexism" (BS), and "hostile sexism" (HS). BS is all the ways women are put on pedestals and perceived as weaker and in need of special care (I'd also call that BS, though perhaps to stand for something else); whereas, HS is the more obvious derogatory portrayals of women. Needless to say, the study found that women supported the gender roles much more when the behaviors were what might be categorized as BS.

That some women support their own subjugation is hardly new, of course.

In 1895, when suffragist Frances Willard wrote *How I Learned to Ride the Bicycle*, in which Willard theorized that the skills and independence needed to ride a bicycle couldn't help but spill over into a woman's personal life, her publication inspired moral outrage in quite a few women who objected strongly to her ideas. I love this line from an editorial at the time: "At least half the interest of one sex in another arises from their respective dependent and protective positions. When a lady velocipedes, she destroys all this kind of subtle interest."

Velocipede. What a word that is. I think I'll challenge myself to work it into daily conversation.

Outraged by the outrage, fellow suffragist Susan B. Anthony (yes, I'm partial to Ms. B.), stepped into the fray, writing in her periodical—aptly called *Revolution*, "Bicycling has done more to emancipate women than any one thing in the world . . . A woman awheel is the picture of untrammeled womanhood." (And yes, I'm clearly partial to this quote, too.) Rock on, Susan and Frances. We need to remember how hard you fought for us more often.

"We still believe to some extent in the gentility of the feminine ideal, that we are the fairer sex, and therefore passive, demure, accommodating, and submissive."

Because if we dig into our psyches and uncover the invisible-to-the-naked-eye social conditioning we've all undergone, most of us will see that we were raised to believe that men are the stronger sex. We still believe to some extent in the gentility of the feminine ideal, that we are the fairer sex, and therefore passive, demure, accommodating, and submissive. Bring on the fainting couch, I'm feeling poorly. All of which brings with it the flip side of what the stereotype says we are *not*—bold, fierce, strong, and independent. Those are masculine qualities, and woe-betide the "shrew" who exhibits them in her personality. Time for some taming. I have often encountered men who comment on my strong opinions as surprising in a woman.

And the comment always fosters a moment of self-doubt, *Am I not feminine enough?* Is it un-demure to feel passionately about, say, the treatment of animals by the food industry?

While for the most part, the 1950s ideal has been relegated to slick television shows (I admit to a serious *Mad Men* addiction), and women are getting closer to equal treatment in their careers, sexism is still deeply rooted in sports—despite Title IX. Remember, 1984 is when women were first allowed to compete in the Olympic marathon. Until then the marathon had been off-limits to us, for fear of jostling our wombs. I'll leave it to others to puzzle over why the womb (inside our bodies, surrounded by other cushy organs) is so much more prone to getting shaken up than a man's testes, which are, how shall I say it, more *vulnerable.*

Yes, men have the Y chromosome, which generally enables them to pack on bigger, stronger muscles, but that doesn't mean women aren't strong in their own right—hello Serena and Venus Williams, Mia Hamm, Lynn Hill, Paula Radcliffe, me, and you.

Women don't have to beat men outright at their own race to prove their strength. Biology is stacked against us on that score. The challenge we face is the attitudes and beliefs that men (and women!) have about men's athletic superiority and how women's athleticism ought to be expressed when we meet on the road, in the pool, on the court, in the ring, on the wall or slope, or . . . you get the picture.

When Marta, the former downhill ski racer, was in law school training for a marathon, she did a few training runs with a man who was a fellow law student. Although they were compatible in their training, speed-wise, he made it clear as the marathon approached that he was running his own race; that they shouldn't expect to see each other at the start or finish line.

"He assumed he would beat me and that if I ran with him it would slow him down," she says. "He said we'd connect after the race at the marathon party I was hosting. I didn't really think much about what he said. I figured we'd see soon enough how the race went." Well what do you know . . . as Marta crossed the finish line and stopped to catch her wind, who did she see pushing hard to the finish line about three-hundred yards behind her? Her fellow student.

"Once he got over his surprise, he was totally fine with it," she says. For their wedding three years later, their parents bought each of them a traditional marathon memento: crystal apples with their finish times engraved—3:41 and 3:42.

I once asked my friend Zach how he would feel if his then-girlfriend, now wife, beat him at one of their sports. "That would never happen," he said, cool as a cucumber, as if what I'd said hardly

"They didn't want to be 'chicked,' as in, beaten up the climb by a girl."

merited a second thought. He wasn't being cocky. His wife is slower than him. But it was interesting how firmly entrenched his certainty was. Like many men, he simply believes that his relatively superior male strength will automatically equate to better speed and endurance. And because of this belief, some men may feel compelled to prove it—whether they're conscious of it or not—because our culture tells us that the opposite is emasculating. Remember the men climbing Tuckerman's Ravine with Joelle? They didn't want to be "chicked," as in, beaten up the climb by a girl.

When our tire-changing Texan, Rebecca, is out on the trails with one of her male running partners and she feels like the two of them are running in sync, he'll sometimes make a point of letting her know that he's actually slowing down for her. She's not, in fact, keeping up with *him*. I wondered why she chose to run with him, since that sounded annoying to me.

"I don't feel competitive with him," she says, "even though it seems like he's being competitive with me. I run with him and other men I know because they've set the standard for things I want to accomplish in running, so it spurs me on. And I like them, even if they say dumb things sometimes."

Laura Fields, an attorney and runner in her midthirties, deals with a similar issue, but with her husband. All too often, going out for a mountain bike ride, ski, or run can feel less like a companionable outing and more like a competition between them. "He'd rather cough up a lung than be beaten by me," she says. "It's annoying, especially when I'm feeling good about, say, my run, he'll keep trying to race me into the ground, even though I run way more than he does. I just try to stay inside my own workout and forget about whatever he's up to. I think it must be exhausting to be him, always needing to beat me," she adds, with a rueful smile.

Laura's husband is hardly unique. His behavior is driven (just as mine was on the mountain) by the pervasive stereotype that men are simply always better athletes, with no accounting for individual circumstances. Just the other night I was in a restaurant and heard this exchange between two men:

Man One: "Are you skiing tomorrow?"

Man Two: "Not really. I'm skiing with a girl."

Yes, I know, that was a joke, but come *on*. A more tolerant friend of mine said, "He didn't mean it to be mean-spirited. I bet if you confronted him, he'd be embarrassed and take it back."

I like how she thinks. Me, I'm ready to rush to the defense of women with my metaphorical guns blazing. She's so much more reasonable, seeing the unwitting cultural conditioning in the com-

"'Female strength is, even yet, seditious. It can make men squirm.'"

ment, recognizing the power of knowing that their attitudes are antiquated. As she says, "When we participate in sports, as we get stronger, we're often breaking mini glass ceilings." And as my friend often demonstrates in her own actions, the better part of valor is to rise above the misconceptions, to be secure in our own strength and power, and to demonstrate the fallacy of the stereotypes. How?—by running like girls, right through those glass ceilings.

As Natalie Angier wrote in her classic book, *Woman: An Intimate Geography*, "Female strength is, even yet, seditious. It can make men squirm."

OUR SEDITIOUS STRENGTH

Women are a force to be reckoned with, not junior members of the sports club of life, waiting for men to give them full membership.

Still, not everyone's up to speed on this yet. We've come a long way, baby—as the old Virginia Slims ad used to say—but there's still some distance to cover.

In 1992, UCLA professors Brian Whipp and Susan Ward published an article in the journal *Nature* titled "Will Women Soon Outrun Men?" Their research suggested that if trends in women's versus men's speed improvements of the prior seventy years continued, women runners would catch up to and possibly surpass male runners in the next fifty years. What is most interesting is not the article itself, which has since been the subject of many counter-studies (none of which have completely debunked the point made), but the reaction from the male running community. Prominent men in the running community, who shall remain nameless because I'm going to give them the benefit of the doubt and assume they'd be embarrassed to see their arrogant words in print so many years later (now that they hopefully know better), were quoted as saying things like, "Women will never run as fast as men! Never, ever, ever!" and "ludicrous," and "ridiculous."

Granted, these men were from the generation weaned on the Boston Marathon as an all-male race until the mid-'70s. I suspect when they began running they still wore white cotton tube socks. And they predated Title IX by a long shot. We know that Title IX rocked the male-dominated sports world. Not only were women required to be recognized as worthy enough to compete, but the new law said that boys and men *had* to let them compete, like it or not. Unfortunately, Title IX was not, as we saw earlier, the ultimate panacea. No law can guarantee a change in attitude.

Just ask Virginia, a sixth-degree black belt and karate teacher. Until she was eighteen, most boys weren't sure what to make of her.

"Sure, they thought my martial arts training was cool, but they saw me more as a 'guy' friend than a possible girlfriend," she recalls. "Ergo, I had very few dates in high school." She's married now, to a man who she says was willing to date her in spite of her martial arts experience. But that's not the end of the challenges she's had to face with men in the karate world.

Once, a new male student said he wouldn't spar with her because he didn't want to "hurt a girl." Unfortunately for him, he didn't have a choice—she was the instructor; he *had* to spar with her. During the match, Virginia lightly tapped him in his vulnerable areas, as is customary, to let him know when he had mistakenly left openings. When she tapped him in the groin, he became angry.

"He immediately stopped sparring with me and walked away toward the head instructor, complaining that I had kicked him 'where it counts.' The head instructor repeated my own instructions about the groin being a legal target and tried to explain to the student that he should listen to my advice if he wanted to become a better martial artist," says Virginia. "But he didn't like the instructor's response and literally walked out. We never saw him again."

Virginia didn't accept, excuse, or ignore the male student's attitude. She took the more productive route of proving her worth.

Pat Griffin, college coach and author, wrote about the pleasure she took in doing just that when she played baseball better than a boy: "I learned to appreciate the special satisfaction there is in beating a guy who considers himself my better just because he's a guy."

You go girls! Yet Pat and Virginia are special women. Not all of us can out-pitch, out-spar, out-run, out-ski, or out-*anything* the men we encounter in our lives. Putting too much stress on trying to

"Our mission, should we choose to accept it, is to do our best, and let our accomplishments speak for themselves. . . "

beat the boys can backfire, undermining our own sense of achievement and ability. Our mission, should we choose to accept it, is to do our best, and let our accomplishments speak for themselves—whether the audience is our own selves or others, including men.

Easier said than done, of course.

Katrine, the triathlete in the advertising business, has been with her husband for five years. In fact, he got her into serious running and doing triathlons. Now they're both equally dedicated athletes. In the beginning, Katrine was very competitive with her mate. Because he was faster than she was, Katrine had trouble seeing her own accomplishments as worthy. She would drive herself to train at least as much as him, if not more. After a few years of living in the swirl of her own *self-generated* competitiveness, she realized that she

"He was already deeply impressed by her athletic talent, and wondered why she wasn't as amazed by her own self as he was."

needed to, as she says, "beat that beast" out of her mind. She needed to be comfortable with—no, *more* than that—she needed to be happy and proud of her own accomplishments and stop comparing herself to her speedier mate, who, incidentally, had some biology on his side. He agreed. He was already deeply impressed by her athletic talent, and wondered why she wasn't as amazed by her own self as he was. Katrine needed a couple of years to grow into her new athletic self, to experience, for example, racing with other women whose strength she admired, only to realize, "Hey, I'm just as strong as they are." Now she's evolved a better balance in her attitude. She doesn't need to compare herself to her husband; her strength stands on its own.

A close male friend I love running with is, as many of our mutual friends say, "a gifted athlete." He makes running look effortless. Yet sometimes a little part of me wants to point out, "Hey, he *is* gifted, and he *is* faster than me, but I actually do better among my peers. Notice *me*." Now who needs to change *her* attitude and get a little more centered in her *own* accomplishments? Why can't it be enough that I know what I've achieved?

There is, after all, an important difference between relative and absolute performance—just because you beat me, doesn't mean you *beat* me. Someone (a man for example) might be absolutely faster than us, but relatively not. There are methods of "leveling the field" statistically, both for age and gender, called "normalizing" the scores. And when scores are normalized, the picture might look awfully different. One measure, for example, is how you perform within your cohort; that is, in the group of people who are most "like" you—your gender and age group, in other words. How I stack up absolutely against men my age is far less relevant than how I stack up among women my age. And even then, what matters is that we do the best by ourselves. I find peace in my athletic pursuits when I stop measuring myself against others and measure myself instead against my own goals and needs at any given time.

Then again, sometimes women *are* simply better than men under certain conditions, particularly when it comes to endurance.

 "Apparently, 50 percent or less of the men who start the Leadville 100 actually finish, but 90 percent or more of the women *do*."

Case in point. More women finish the Leadville 100 race every year than men. Let me back up and give you some context. I came across the Leadville statistic in Christopher McDougall's book, *Born to Run,* which includes stories about this grueling one-hundred-mile trail race held each year in Colorado. Apparently, 50 percent or less of the men who start the Leadville 100 actually finish, but 90 percent or more of the women *do*.

The Leadville phenomenon is backed up by studies, which show that as distances increase, women's performance improves relative to men of similar speed at the shorter distances. A South African study looked at why women slowed down less than men over the long haul and could not find a strong physiological reason, though the study theorized that estrogen ameliorated the breakdown of muscle that naturally occurs in long races. Other studies have suggested that men, fueled by testosterone, rush out of the starting gate too fast and burn themselves out more often than women. Or maybe it's all those strong gorgeous women runners in the races with them. Because other studies have shown that a man's testosterone level elevates in the presence of a pretty woman, causing him to take greater physical risks than he would if he was just hanging out with the guys.

> "No slowing down, playing weak, or pretending fragility to placate others."

Whatever the reason, women clearly have what it takes to go the distance. We always knew that, of course, and as we move into the future, we will grow a critical mass of strong women who will set the standards for all of us—as the norm, *not* the exception.

We need to be true to our nature. No slowing down, playing weak, or pretending fragility to placate others. We need to let our strength shine. Authenticity. Integrity. Honesty. *These* are the qualities worth cultivating. *That's* what it means to run like a girl.

WE'RE *WOMEN* NOT WII GAMES

Unfortunately, regardless of whether or not a woman is stronger than her man, her sheer athleticism can itself create friction.

When Helen Bollinger, a real estate agent and runner now in her late fifties, met her third husband, she was a serious athlete. She ran ten miles a day, did multisport races, and in the winter would go for long backcountry ski adventures. Her new husband wanted her to teach him how to run, but he never wanted to run farther than a mile. Helen went from ten miles a day to one mile a day of running.

"I allowed him to control my participation in sports because I thought it was my duty to keep him happy. When our daughter was born, if I tried to head out for a longer run, he would say, 'But what if the baby cries?' Well, that would stop me in my tracks. I

> "Sometimes it seems like men think we're part of the Wii game of life, and they have control of the joystick."

didn't want to ask too much of him. So I'd abandon my plans to put in a few extra miles."

It's been four years since Helen ended that twenty-plus year marriage.

"I now see all the ways I let him redefine me as an athlete," she says. At the age of fifty-eight, she's rediscovering the sports that gave her so much joy.

Helen's situation is not unique. Sometimes it seems like men think we're part of the Wii game of life, and they have control of the joystick.

Mary, the teacher and coach, gave up volleyball for a time because her boyfriend. "P," as she calls him, had surgery on his shoulder, preventing him from playing volleyball, so he didn't want to watch her play. She said it made him depressed to be reminded of what he couldn't do.

"It was all about him," Mary says. "I thought that to be supportive I should do the things he wanted. So I stopped playing volleyball and actually started smoking because *he* was a smoker. I thought that smoking and doing no sports was something we could share. In hindsight, I know, it was crazy on my part."

Fast forward a year later and Mary is an out of shape smoker and feeling restless with her state of affairs. A friend invites her to run a 5k with her, and one thing leads to another. Before long, Mary and her friend are signed up to run a half marathon together.

"I began training for the half marathon, and suddenly there *I* was again," she recalls. "During those runs, my mind cleared . . . I would think about my relationship with P, and I realized that I had lost myself."

On more than one occasion her boyfriend told her she was "crazy" for wanting to run a half marathon. On race day, guess who didn't show up?

"Her boyfriend told her she was 'crazy' for wanting to run a half marathon. On race day, guess who didn't show up?"

"Not long after that I broke up with him—something he had once told me I would never have the strength to do." Turns out Mary was *that* strong, and more. She walked away from the control *and* the condescension.

Like Kelly, the coach and professional triathlete, says, "When a man condescends to me in my sports, I simply walk away, because if they are so full of themselves to think that women are less capable, then in my opinion they are lacking self-confidence and they need to get in touch with reality."

We may feel challenged by the outdated attitudes and behaviors of some men, but in the end we have the power to filter out what doesn't do us good, what doesn't add to our well-being, or our sense of self. Coping with less-than-supportive messages that might come our way is simply an opportunity to reinforce our psychological strength and determination. As one of my meditation teachers, Kadam Morten, says, "The challenges in life are all opportunities to purify our karma by teaching us the practices of forbearance, patience, and perseverance."

When Michelle, the founder of the Society for Martial Arts Instruction, started practicing Tae Kwon Do, she did so with her husband. By her estimate, if she was putting 150 percent into her practice, then her husband was putting in about 20 percent. And yet the sensei treated her and her husband the same. In fact, at one point, she says, her sensei explicitly said, "I won't test you ahead of your husband." For years Michelle's progress in karate (she switched from Tae Kwon Do) was held back by her husband's 20 percent efforts. She was not allowed to test until he was ready for each successive level, which was well after she was ready. Finally, when Michelle earned her black belt, her sensei told her she could now test alone. (In martial arts, by the way, a black belt is only the beginning, then comes the hardest challenges, the different degrees of the black belt.)

So why did Michelle stay? Many of us would have quit in indignation, and who could blame such a response? "I kept asking myself, why am I here? Is it for me or for them? And the answer was—for me. I stuck to the practice for *me*."

That didn't always make putting up with the chauvinistic behavior easier, of course. She had to recommit to her practice often and remind herself why she was there. She had to breathe through the ancient Japanese traditions, which, like so many Western traditions, are poorly adapted to women.

"I don't blame them anymore," Michelle says. "They just don't know what to do with us." By which she means "us women."

Finally testing for her black belt was only the beginning for Michelle. Once she had achieved that important level, she struck out on her own and created her own martial arts dojo. A space where women are respected equals. A space where what women bring to martial arts—their natural lightness, their flexibility of mind and body, and their instinct to de-escalate—are incorporated into the practice.

Michelle's sensei might have controlled the pace at which she tested, but Michelle was able to relax into the pace and find her own rhythm, one that suited her needs. Men may try to control us. Our task is to take what we need from the behavior and sidestep the rest. We are only controlled if we let ourselves be.

If a man can't take a woman who excels in karate, or volleyball, or indeed any sport, that's *his* issue, not ours. Focusing on our own desires and goals when it comes to our sports can be a challenge if the men around us aren't as supportive as they might be. But then again, if someone close to us isn't supportive of one of our passions in life, what does that say about our ability to have an honest and fulfilling relationship with that person, let alone ourselves (after all we picked the relationship)? Know our worth. It's our reserve of confidence when external discouragement threatens our equilibrium, when someone tries to control our strength.

Of course, not all male control is nefarious. Life is necessarily a dance of give and take, sometimes we lead and sometimes we follow. Laura, the founder of Team Lipstick and a former competitive

"Life is necessarily a dance of give and take, sometimes we lead and sometimes we follow."

ballroom dancer, says the "lead/follow" of dance, when done well, is a profound nonverbal language to experience. The best lead partners, as she says, "have a nice accent" in the language of dance. The accent is what matters, whether we're leading or being led. The wrong accent can upset the harmonious flow of the dance of life—too much control will be stiff and awkward, jerking a person around the floor. Watch out for those toes.

When it comes to the men in our lives, it sometimes feels easier to let them lead than to let them know when they've trod on our toes. This is particularly true when the control comes in subtle forms, such as when men feel compelled to offer well meaning but unsolicited advice. Because once again, most men—whether conditioned to feel this way or not—assume they corner the market on athletic expertise.

I'M DOING JUST FINE, THANK YOU

For years, my partner, a cross-country ski racer in college, used to offer frequent suggestions on how I might improve my cross-country skiing technique. Apart from "hiking" on cross-country skis through the woods with my parents as a child, I had no idea what I was doing when I first began. I didn't even know there were two types of cross-country skiing, each requiring a different set of skis.

Classic, or striding, is the type of cross-country skiing most of us are familiar with. It's where you keep your skis parallel and glide down carved-out tracks in the snow. Skate skiing is very different. It requires shorter skis, an outward-arcing ice skating motion, and it's done on the kind of wide, corduroy-groomed trails we're familiar with from downhill skiing. Skate skiing is faster than classic, but arguably less elegant. Particularly when it's me on them without a clue about what to do.

My novice status, coupled with my partner's decades of serious experience, naturally led to a teacher-student dynamic. I was eager to improve my technique, but I chafed against the power structure, wanting to enjoy the sport on equal footing, even if not at equal speed. So my partner's technique tips, while helpful, were a constant reminder of my weaknesses and his strengths, so that I felt a constant low-level of frustration with him—and even more with myself—every time I wore my skis. It was discouraging to feel that, no matter how hard I tried, I could never catch up to his years of ski racing.

Not one to give up easily, especially after too many semi-agitated years doing this, I finally signed up for an all-women's ski clinic. Participating in the clinic provided me with a degree of comfort in my own skill and knowledge, which made it much easier to accept his advice more gracefully, and without feeling condescended to. Not that my partner's advice was ever intended that way. I just had to gain confidence in my own abilities, to hear the correct "accent."

It can be hard ignoring a man's advice, particularly from a husband, lover, boyfriend, or significant other, but just like any other influence in our lives, we need to find that peaceful place where we take in what is useful and let the rest go.

Of course, it's *much* easier when the men are strangers. When Justine, who's in the film business, is at the gym, she says, "Men frequently approach me to give me advice on my workouts. As in, 'you should be doing it this way.' Did I ask for their advice?" Justine has a demanding job in a cutthroat industry, so she has no problem ignoring unsolicited advisors.

One of the reasons men seem to be freer with their advice is simply because they're often more experienced in the sports. After all, despite Title IX, men still begin participating in sports earlier than girls.

 "Man says, 'It's easy.' Man says, 'I'll show you how.'"

Here's one dynamic many of us will be familiar with. Man takes woman out for a too-challenging run, ride, ski, or other sport that's difficult to master without prior experience or instruction. Man says, "It's easy." Man says, "I'll show you how." Right before we fall flat on our faces. I'm not alone here, right?

In a similar vein, there's the "charity rides," as Nora, the former figure skater, calls them. That's when her husband, a much faster cyclist than she is, rides with her on his "slow days," all the while riding comfortably within his limit, so he has lots of spare wind to dispense advice. "Of course, I'll never ride faster than him. When he rides with me it's about him controlling my workout."

From bike maintenance to race strategy, men may want to counsel us, whether we've asked for it or not. Because it happens, we don't always need it. Men are *not* always the experts.

I once competed in a half Ironman race with my friend Andrea. Her husband had come to spectate and cycle alongside the race. When I finished, flushed with the thrill and surprise of being in third place among all women, Andrea's husband was nowhere to be seen. The plan was that he'd meet us there to watch our finish. Some minutes later, as I stood in line for the massage table, I spotted him heading toward the finish line. I called out to him, excited to share my news with someone. "You're done?" He asked. I happily told him that I was not only done, but had finished quite respectably. "That's great," he said, adding without a pause for breath, "Next time, you really need to get tri-bars."

 "I wanted a grace period to bask in my fleeting glory before getting advice about how I could do better. . . . "

Granted, he's a gifted cyclist, but he's not a *triathlete*—and I wanted a grace period to bask in my fleeting glory before getting advice about how I could do better, if only I did this or that. No grace period. In the end it doesn't matter. I was happy with my result, and no amount of ex post facto advice could change what I'd accomplished. And anyway, it was up to me to provide myself the grace period I wanted.

Enough about me though, back to me. Speaking of grace periods. . . .

Only a week after the all women's ski clinic I mentioned, my partner complimented my improved technique. Grace period: thirty seconds. Then he suggested that now I should try working on a difficult technique called "V2," which, because I'd always found it complicated, not to mention ultra-exhausting, I'd avoided for the whole decade I'd been skiing. V2 is the power stroke in skate skiing, like the biggest gear on your bike. Sure it's good to have if you're going to go really fast, but it's not strictly necessary. But fresh off my ski clinic, buoyed by my newfound confidence, it turns out I didn't *need* a grace period. More, I truly understood that his advice had everything to do with his confidence in my ability, and nothing to do with condescension. I spent the next week forcing myself to

"[I]nstead of resenting my partner's advice, I was grateful that he'd given me the extra push."

master the V2. At first I thought I might blow open from exhaustion, literally—heart exploded to shreds, making a sticky red mess on the nice white ski trail—then I began to dial it in.

The first time I skied around the whole of a particular one-mile loop comfortably, without once straying from my V2, was a thrill. It was empowering. And instead of resenting my partner's advice, I was grateful that he'd given me the extra push.

Because when it comes down to it, the spirit in which we receive advice is so much more important than the spirit in which it's given, whether it comes from our male partners or not.

WOMEN PLUS MEN EQUALS TWICE AS MANY FRIENDS

In fact, the spirit in which we do *anything* is really the bottom line.

When my brother Noah and I have access to the outdoors together, we usually find some way to make a ten-course meal of it. Some weekends are so jam-packed, it feels like a full session of summer camp. Both days are filled with more outdoor activities than some people do in a year, or at least it seems like it. During one memorable trip, we were driving full bore into the Adirondacks, on our way to climb Rogers Rock, when the canoe lashed to the top of our truck started to slip, threatening to launch right off the back. We retied the boat more securely and drove at a more sedate pace to our destination, periodically breaking into giggles as we contemplated the potential disaster we'd averted.

Why, you may wonder, did we have a canoe when we were going climbing? Well this particular climb required a canoe. As in, we had to canoe in to the rock face, pull the boat onto a little ledge, and then climb up from there. The day was magnificent, and we couldn't resist a little swim after the climb, not to mention that we'd warmed up for the day with a bit of a trail run. By the time we got home, and the canoe was safely stored back on its dock, we had barely enough energy to boil water for pasta and flop down to watch a silly movie before bed, before the *next* activity-filled day.

 "[D]espite all the fraught and friction that can infect the sports relations between women and men, we can also be friends on the playing field."

This is my long-winded way of saying that, despite all the fraught and friction that can infect the sports relations between women and men, we can also be friends on the playing field. Women plus men makes twice as many friends.

Take Kristen, for example. She's a fly-fishing manufacturer's representative and runner who took up fly-fishing when she started dating her boyfriend, now husband. Fly-fishing, as she points out, is one of the few sports that's easy for people of different skill levels to do together. Because it's done in parallel, there is no need to "keep up" with the person you're fishing with. So the dynamic of competition is eliminated and no one needs to worry about holding another person back.

Yet even if speed or strength might notionally matter, not everything needs to become a competition, a case of who's-bigger-stronger.

Despite her petite, five-foot-three-inch frame, Michelle Prior regularly rides with a group of hardcore male mountain bikers. She's not their token woman. She just happens to be friends with the boys, and the only woman who hits the trail with them to ride hard and have fun. A midforties single mother and avid runner from California, Michelle says, "The rides are never about who maneuvers the best around the technical spots, it's all about the thrill of the descent. We've *all* taken spills. We all have scars. Skill, experience, quick thinking . . . a bit of fearlessness, all determine how well we do on the trail, not our gender. Really," she says, "it's about hanging out with people I like."

Skill, experience, quick thinking, and friendship. That sounds like a gender leveling sport, which sounds an awful lot like rock climbing—if you throw in grace and elegance as well. Rock climbing is, by many people's assessment, the ultimate equal opportunity sport. Because unlike so many other sports, it doesn't necessarily favor bulk, speed, strength, or height. In fact, bulk and strength can sometimes work against a person. First, because they have to haul all that weight up the rock face (rock climbing is more about strength-to-weight ratio than how purely strong you are); and, probably more important, because someone strong may be inclined to rely on their brute strength through the easier bits of a climb and end up in trouble because they're *not* climbing like a girl, with finesse and balance.

So if you're looking for the possibility of absolute and relative parity in a sport, it might be time to strap on a harness. Unfortunately, other than climbing, and possibly a few other select sports like horseback riding, figure skating, and ski jumping, the biological fact is that, on average, men will have a strength and size advantage over us, which as we've seen, also means that men often believe they are better than us at whatever our sport is, just by virtue of the fact that they are men. In individual sports we can learn

 "From soccer and basketball to dodge ball and adventure races, countless men and women play side-by-side without a spark of gender friction."

to tune out the male superiority complex, but on a team, that gets more difficult. We don't often get to choose every single one of our teammates. On the other hand, there's something about batting for the same team, literally, that fosters camaraderie—especially when you're doing it for fun. From soccer and basketball to dodge ball and adventure races, countless men and women play side-by-side without a spark of gender friction. I'll say nothing about other kinds of sparks. Suffice to say here that more than one relationship has bloomed over a nice sweaty bout of athletics. Why does it work?—competition, or rather the lack thereof. When the worst the loser suffers is spotting the winners for pizza and beer, and when the sports are a social experience above all, fun happens.

The added bonus is that sometimes when women play with men, they have the opportunity to change their worldview—*both* of theirs—just that little bit, undo a fraction of all that social conditioning.

As an adventure mentor for families, Laural spent a year playing in a recreational male hockey league. Without size in her favor, Laural relied on her speed, tenacity, and ability to hunker down really low when someone was barreling at her from the other end of the rink. Earning the men's respect took time, but her reward finally came in the form of an opposing player turning to his teammate and saying, "I didn't notice she was a girl." But what truly sealed her acceptance as part of the team happened in the co-ed locker room, of all places. One of the men momentarily forgot that Laural was a woman and, without thinking, dropped his towel post-shower.

"It was funny," she recalls, "and I took it as the highest praise possible, because in that moment he saw me as a teammate, just like everyone else."

In an aggressive, highly "male" sport, Laural had proven that what's under the towel is less important than whose wearing the

 "Laural had proven that what's under the towel is less important than whose wearing the skates."

skates. She had shown her teammates a whole new way to look at women, as one of the guys.

Although perhaps not as overtly aggressive as hockey, golf is another sport that's a largely male, dare I say "white," sport. Even now, some golf courses are closed to women during busy weekends. Turns out, says Christie Howard, who handles corporate partnerships for the Ladies Pro Golf Association (LPGA), when women get up the gumption to go out on the course, the biggest surprise is that often the men don't play quite as good a game as they've talked.

Jane Blalock, a top pro golfer from 1969 to 1986, agrees. "Women," she says, "are always thinking, 'I'm not good enough,' whereas men will go out to play golf even if they've never played before. Women have no idea how pitiful men's golf games often are. The men are out there to have fun, to socialize, and to hang out with clients. Women want to have studied and practiced and be good before they feel comfortable joining."

Jane, who discovered her natural talent for golf while playing whiffle ball as a child, is now working to help women overcome their intimidation and get out on the course. It began after she retired from seventeen years of professional golf and took up financial advising for Merrill Lynch. As she progressed in her career, she noticed that golf increased her access to new business. She also noticed that the only other woman typically at the golf event was working behind the beverage cart. She decided it was time to help women penetrate this traditionally "inner sanctum" of business, so she started the Jane Blalock Company. Her strategy? To teach women to play golf well enough that they feel confident to not only get out on the course but to also participate in corporate, industry, and charity golf events.

"When I teach golf, I'm teaching strategic planning, focus, how to win and lose, and the perseverance to dismiss a loss and learn from the negative." As Jane says, "I'm an optimist and a realist, and I don't give up on things."

Still, even when we're "just one of the guys," women among men often find it most effective to maintain some gender differences.

As captain of four-person adventure race teams where she's the only woman, Rebecca Rusch says she tends to use a bit more finesse than guys when she's delivering her team instructions—from crossing a river to scaling a wall. Given the extreme athleticism of the men on these teams, not to mention their skill and confidence, she presents her opinions on strategies for particular race challenges in a *gentler* manner than her male counterparts might present them.

"I don't just shout them out," she says. And by that she means as *men* are likely to do. What might be thought of as forceful and commanding from a man is often thought of as strident from a woman. Given her many wins, Rebecca clearly hits the right notes to inspire a team into winning action.

Women like Rebecca and Laural, along with so many others, are proving that despite all the social conditioning that might be stacked against us, women and men can play well together. And once we find out how fun it can be, on both sides, there's no turning back.

MORE THAN A FEW GOOD MEN

We know we can have fun together, but sometimes we need to figure it out a bit before we get it just right.

I still think about Kilimanjaro, even though it was twenty years ago. I don't resent my former husband for what *I* did. I disappointed myself by not understanding what was important to me, what I needed for myself. About a decade later I got a second chance to revisit my own social conditioning. Different man, different challenge. I was doing my first half Ironman—that's a 1.2-mile swim, a fifty-six-mile bike, and a 13.1-mile run (i.e., a half marathon). In triathlon lingo the race is called a "70.3," as in the total of all the miles covered.

"[A]head of me, in a ripple of heat puffing skyward from the dark pavement, I saw the man who was my life partner."

I was nine miles into the run—the final leg of the race—when ahead of me, in a ripple of heat puffing skyward from the dark pavement, I saw the man who was my life partner. Could I pass him, or should I slow down? Until that moment he had beaten me in every kind of race we had ever done together. I realized it was important to me to do my best—for *me.* I wanted to see what I was capable of. Despite the heat and limited access to water on the course, I felt strong. But as I got closer, I could see he wasn't feeling the same. I felt my pace slowing. What to do? I could hang back and finish just behind him. I could catch up to him and run with him, at his pace. Or I could run my own race. Many of you might be thinking—why was that even a choice? In the middle of a race, I had come smack up against my own socially conditioned response about gender roles and expectations. But unlike with Kilimanjaro, this time I succeeded in censoring my internal agita. I trusted that my partner respected me and was secure enough in his own extraordinary talents to accept my strength. He did. As I ran past, he gave me a shout-out and we high-fived. That race was the first time I finished before him, but not the last.

He still thinks it's crazy that I questioned making the decision to pass him. To him, my strength was a given. I made assumptions about the dynamics of our competition because he was a man, without taking into account what *kind* of man—the kind who wants his partner to shine at whatever she does, even if she happens to be doing it better than him that day.

 "[N]ot all men are threatened by women who are more talented athletes than they are."

Nothing happens in a vacuum, and certainly not gender-balance issues in sports. We women can also be complicit in perpetuating the antiquated status quo of "men as superior athletes." Guilty as charged. On the other side, not all men are threatened by women who are more talented athletes than they are. To wit, my own experience. Nor do men necessarily feel the need to compete with the women in their lives, or indeed *any* woman.

Robin, the former Wall Street broker, is married to an avid golfer who took up running, something that's always been Robin's "thing."

"He'd always supported my running," says Robin, "but until recently, he didn't really run himself. He's not as fast as I am, and we don't train together. But that's not an issue with him. He's doing it for himself because he's inspired by how much I love it, and the fact that it keeps me in good shape."

Often the opposite happens. For many of the women I interviewed, the sports they've chosen to pursue developed from their relationship(s) with men—fathers, brothers, a boyfriend, or husband. Three cheers for the positive effects of men in our athletic lives.

Take Jo, from the district attorney's office. She took up running in 1968 (a time when very few women ran competitively), because "husband number one" thought she ought to, and *she* thought she ought to do what he wanted. He gave her a running book that said her hair would become thicker and her nails would grow faster. At first, Jo had to lie down after the first quarter mile. Then she got hooked. She'd wear her sneakers to bed to make getting up in the morning easier. Next, her husband said she had to compete in races. She thought her day job was competitive enough. Still, she did the races. Why? At first it was because "husband number one's" challenges and demands made her mad, an incentive to do better in every race. She transformed her anger into crossing the finish line of nine New York Marathons, joyful experiences, every one. As she says, "I cried every time I crossed the finish line."

She's married to husband number two now, and he doesn't demand she take up the activities he chooses, nor does he make her mad.

"I'm grateful to husband number one for getting me into running. Next to work and family, it's one of the most important things in my life."

> "[T]he whole creates a gorgeous quilt of the extraordinary richness that men and women bring to each other's lives."

In the end, regardless of whether we feel challenged, coerced, offended, or cowed by the attitudes and behaviors of some men, our job is to filter out what doesn't enhance our well-being or sense of self and embrace the healthy, positive relationships we *do* have with men. Ultimately, the sometimes sticky, hopefully more often lovely, relationships we foster with men in sports depend on *our* attitudes as much as anything else. We embrace the good with the bad, yin and yang, Mars and Venus. And when we do, the whole creates a gorgeous quilt of the extraordinary richness that men and women bring to each other's lives.

The ride up Col des Fourches in the south of France is an unrelenting ten-kilometer climb. We've fueled up on croissant and brioche at the bakery before starting the ascent. I'm riding with my partner and my youngest brother, two of the treasured men in my life. At the top we take a break under a tree with a trunk so fat my arms can't fit around it. Draped over our handlebars with our tongues hanging out, like dogs enjoying the breeze out of the car window. Dappled sunlight ripples through the awning of leaves. Tar patches on the road bubble in the heat. When we've caught our breath, we nod at each other, smiling, time to go. The descent is thrilling. The rugged road jounces our hands, so that we have to shake them out at intervals, letting go of the brakes for short moments, adding to the reckless excitement of the down. The road is narrow and falls away on our traffic side. There's no guardrail, unless you count the knee-high wildflowers shaking their purple, yellow, and white heads at us as we zoom by. I lose sight of my partner and brother almost immediately. I'm pumping my brakes. They are flying, one chasing the other down the mountain.

My heart catches in my throat for just a moment as I watch them disappear. There goes my life, I think, imagining them careening off into thin air. I'm glad I don't have to watch this part of their ride.

At the bottom they are waiting for me, happily exhilarated. My heart fits itself back into its proper place in my chest. *Safe and sound.* These two men I can't imagine living without. When we're done with our ride we'll go go-karting, then we'll stuff ourselves silly at the dirt-floor restaurant we love.

A perfect day.

CHAPTER 7:

Will You Be My Friend?

"I wonder what Piglet is doing," thought Pooh.
"I wish I were there to be doing it, too."
—Winnie the Pooh

My running partner Tammy and I have been "together" for more than fifteen years. When she deserted me—okay, when she moved out to New Jersey—she insisted that our friendship on the road was too important to give up, so she drives in to the city once a week to meet me for a run in New York's Central Park. There's nothing I can't share with her, and we never run out of topics to talk about. Every time I spot her graceful loping stride as she approaches our appointed meeting spot, I'm grateful to have such a devoted workout mate and friend. She's my ear, my advisor, and my life cheerleader. As a matter of fact, it was she who said to me one day, "When are you going to write about us?" And her question got me thinking. . . .

S ports nourish more than our bodies. They can also feed our human need for companionship—and I mean the type more nurturing than some we saw in the last chapter.

But as we move past our university days, and our so-called "real life" sets in—some version of establishing a career, forming a life partnership, and creating a family—making new friends gets harder. Gone are the days when we spent late afternoons hanging out with friends we'd just made in history class, or at recess, or in the line at the cafeteria. "Let's get together" is made more difficult and complicated by responsibilities and obligations. "There's work tomorrow, so I can't stay out too late" . . . "The laundry really needs to get done (no more taking it home to my parent's house on the weekend)" . . . "What's for dinner (now that ramen noodles no longer suffice for every meal)" . . . "I need to drive carpool for a playdate. . . ."

Wait a minute—just because we're supposedly adults now doesn't mean we can't have and don't *need* playdates, too. Need?— you ask. Studies from every angle have shown the health benefits that friendship has on our ability to cope with life's sometimes devastating setbacks—divorce, job loss, miscarriage, cancer, to name a few biggies. We humans are social animals, literally. We thrive on the positive interaction of relationships with others. I can't count the number of times I've found myself involuntarily beaming as I head home after time spent with a good friend. The smile is simply there on my face, an instinctive reaction to my feeling of well-being.

> **"'What better way to get to know someone than to test your abilities together, to be daring and sweaty and exhausted together?'"**

As hard as it can be to make new friends as life accelerates, wonderfully for us, sports can be one of the most profound sources of new connections with others.

As former professional basketball player Mariah Burton Nelson says, "What better way to get to know someone than to test your abilities together, to be daring and sweaty and exhausted together?"

OUR FAITHFUL MUSKETEERS

Countless precious friendships can bloom on the trails, mountain slopes, basketball courts, and myriad other places we actively engage with teammates and training partners.

Mary, the president of New York Road Runners, is—surprise (not!)—an avid runner. Like many women, she's balancing her workouts with a demanding career and a family with young children. As Mary says, "My morning runs are a way to squeeze a social life into a very hectic schedule. Often, it's the only time I have to talk to one of my closest friends," who also happens to be her running partner.

Same for Rebecca, the world champion adventure racer. "I need my friends to get me out there. I need people to come out in the rain and for the ridiculously hard workouts." And when she says this, she gives one of her signature gigantic smiles, a glimpse of the high spirit she brings to those workouts with friends. My guess is they are more than happy to join her. "Otherwise," she continues, "the training would be too much of a job." Because unlike most of us, sport *is* Rebecca's job; as a professional adventure racer, she has sponsors to keep happy, which means she needs to participate in a robust roster of races every year, often traveling in the winter (technically her off-season) to races in warmer climes. "Plus, I'd hardly see my friends if we weren't out training together. The social group is a big part of the fun."

Actually, here's research confirming what we have all felt—that working out with friends is more than just good for our souls. A study by scientists at the University of Oxford's Institute of Cognitive and Evolutionary Anthropology found that rowers who worked out together were able to tolerate up to twice as much pain as they could when they trained on their own. So working out with a friend or a team can up your pain threshold, thereby upping the intensity of your training.

If you've worked out with other people, that conclusion is not surprising. My running partner Tammy and I push each other to stay "honest" on our runs and not slack off. On the days I'm flagging, she'll push me to the top of the hills, reminding me how strong I was the week before, and vice versa. We hold each other and ourselves to a higher standard when we're together, without it

"We hold each other and ourselves to a higher standard when we're together, without it being competitive."

being competitive. We want to see what we're capable of, and we want to help each other do the same. I am so proud of my friends when they do well, and the feeling is almost better than when I succeed at something myself. But lest you think my friends and I spend every workout in high gear, that's not so. Some days are for chatting; or as I like to think of it, "chatting with benefits."

"I almost didn't come today," my cycling partner, Rachel, has said to me many a wee early morning in the first pedal strokes of our ride, when we're both feeling still-stoned with sleep. "But then I knew I wanted to see you and catch up," she'll say. I feel the same way.

 "Our workout partner may well be our therapy partner and more, the person with whom we can talk about anything."

There is a unique quality to a relationship built on uninterrupted time with one other person in the focus of a workout: no waiters, no movies, no cell phone calls. There's something about being side-by-side in the parallel play of our individual workouts that can free up our more intimate thoughts, deepening our conversations on the road. Our workout partner may well be our therapy partner and more, the person with whom we can talk about anything.

Colleen, the runner and former Wall Street banker, says that her running friendships are different from other friendships. "They see me un-showered and sweaty and smelly and gross, and presumably they like me anyway," she says. "What is discussed on a run stays on a run. I've told personal things to running buddies that I have not told others, who I've known for years."

Many mountain sports take this closeness one step further. As Lynn, our devotee of the mountains, says, "With activities such as mountaineering there's the element of trust and reliance in potentially dangerous and life-threatening situations that creates a deeper bond."

No doubt that when you're hanging off the end of a rope secured by small pieces of metal stuck into tiny cracks in a rock wall, and your life depends on your partner having placed that "gear" just so, a relationship can feel extra intimate. My brother met his wife climbing, and it's always struck me that they put their lives in each other's hands long before they recorded that reality in a marriage registry.

Yet, my brother and his wife aside, one of the more profound things about our "sports friends" is that to share deep intimacy, they do not have to be our BFFs (that's Best Friends Forever, for those who, like me, aren't hip to the latest acronyms) beyond the sport.

Rebecca, our tire-changing wiz, enjoys the company of many close running friends. "The funny thing is, we are so close, but we've never actually socialized outside of the running atmosphere."

I've had sports friends like that over the years as well, people with whom I share hours of alone time, but never off the road. It's almost as if we don't want to disrupt the magic of our sports friendship by subjecting it to new environments.

Friendships come in different shapes and sizes, from the pale bookworms to the wind-burned jocks. Some of our deepest bonds can be forged when our sports friends cross over and we mesh equally well on the trail or after a movie, in sneakers or strappy heels. What a treasure to have people who inhabit our multiple worlds.

When referring to a new close friend of hers, Nora, the former figure skater, says, "I knew when we started talking about Sylvia Plath while we were on the bike that we were friends beyond sports."

Ginny Redmon, who's been a die-hard runner since 1978, moved to Colorado with her former husband when she was pregnant. "I didn't know a soul. I was lonely, and I cried a lot," she says.

Here she was about to start a family and she had no community of friends to turn to for support. She was fortunate in her pregnancy, and could continue running until close to the end. Running the endless woodsy trails near her new home helped temper her loneliness and angst. Still, she hit the trails alone. Then after the baby was born, she was inspired to sign up for a neighborhood fun run. During the race, she happened to notice a woman pass her who looked to be in her midthirtyish "age group." *Could she be a new friend?* thought Ginny, and she was inspired enough by the idea that when the race was over, she made a point of tracking the woman down.

"I just walked up to Nancy—who was of course a perfect stranger at the time—and asked, 'Will you run with me and be my friend?'" The immediate answer was yes and yes. "Nancy and I still

 "'You name it,' says Ginny, 'we've been there for each other.'"

joke about it to this day." They have remained close friends ever since: through job losses, illness, divorce, the challenges of parenting, and the pleasure of grandchildren. "You name it," says Ginny, "we've been there for each other."

I had occasion to think of Ginny's story when I made a new snow-friend recently. At the end of a women's skate-skiing clinic, I agreed to meet one of the participants the next morning for a "pole-less" ski session. This is where you leave your ski poles in the car, along with the security they provide, and work on your skate-skiing technique without the aid of poles. We spent the morning together, talking nonstop about every topic that came to mind. There wasn't a lull in the conversation, except those enforced by the steepest of the hills—up, as we struggled for breath, and down, as we concentrated on keeping our skis underneath us. I felt like a giddy schoolgirl by the end of our time together. *A new friend! A new friend! A new friend!* I thought to myself.

And she was.

As for all my other friends on the road, old and new, I cherish our time together. They nurture me on the bad days, when I'm tired or sad or frustrated, when I wake up so far on the wrong side of the bed that I wonder if I got out of my own bed or some unhappy doppelganger's bed. They inspire me to reach. "Why not try?" they'll say. "You can," they'll say. "Let's do it together."

A FRIEND IN NEED . . .

As Ginny so astutely pointed out, after that giddy flush of early friendship, the ones that endure are those that survive when life isn't so fresh and fun, when "you name it" happens. These are the friends who give us a hug and a hand and an ear, who scoop us up off the pavement when we're writhing in pain, and then help us heal—not just emotionally, but literally. They help us outrun havoc, even if we end up with a few tear stains on our running shoes. And I know from personal experience that it's possible to cry and run at the same time, but at least I'm running.

Lois, the flight attendant who inspires me with her upbeat attitude, met one of her most cherished friends only six years ago. They met by happenstance, but they were brought together by a shared experience of profound loss.

"I had lost my stepson to suicide, and she had lost her son the same way," Lois told me. "That shared experience cemented our bond, and we helped each other through the grief."

 "'You have to put a lot in your laughter bank to get through the rough patches in life. . .'"

Once they had passed through the worst of the grief, their bond stayed strong through their mutual love of active outdoor adventures. They even started a blog about their escapades under the monikers, "Lotus Blossom and MizzI," writing about everything from their crazy cross-country journeys, to white water rafting and hiking, all undertaken in the highest of spirits, with no purpose but to have fun, and more fun, until . . . well until time runs out.

"You have to put a lot in your laughter bank to get through the rough patches in life," says Lois. "And MizzI helps me do that."

Grief can stop us in our tracks. So much so, that sometimes we need a whole team of friends to help us get on our feet again.

Katie, the triathlete and runner who works in the insurance business, met many of her friends through Team in Training when she was training for her first marathon. For those of you who may not be familiar with the signature purple tops and white lettering, Team in Training is a nonprofit powerhouse that brings together runners, walkers, cyclists, hikers, and triathletes who plan to participate in major athletic events around the world—from marathons and triathlons, to hiking adventures and century rides. Participants join up, train, and compete on behalf of The Leukemia and Lymphoma Society, racing—literally—to raise money to fund research looking for a cure. More than that, many of the participants are either cancer survivors—or family of survivors—or they've lost someone they love to the disease. The team creates a nurturing environment, which, says Katie, can itself be a critical source of healing and strength.

"I'd lost my mother to cancer some years earlier," says Katie, "and I was still grieving." In the beginning, she would show up to team meetings and cry uncontrollably. "I wondered why I ran at all. I had to ask myself, 'Am I having fun?' and at first the answer was 'no.' I realized I was running after something. I was trying to keep my mother."

Ultimately, Katie says, the support and understanding of her teammates helped her work through her grief. Now instead of running after her mother, whom she realizes she can never catch, she runs for a more life-affirming reason: pleasure.

Grief is just one deep manifestation of depression, which is an emotion that can bring us to our knees. The self-destructive behavior that depression can foster runs the gamut from eating a pint of ice cream in front of the open freezer door, to numbing our pain with a salve more toxic: truss my arm and find the vein. Once again, if we're fortunate, we have the right friends who can ride in on a *different* kind of white horse and offer a healthier alternative.

When Carrie, the stand-up comic, first moved to Austin at twenty-four, she knew no one outside the radio-marketing world. "In my limited worldview, I lived the same pretty unhealthy existence as everyone else—drinking and eating too much, and why be active? It was depressing and I was depressed."

As we know, Carrie took up running to mend a broken heart, but the healing went much further. "It changed my worldview. I developed all these great friendships with wonderful fit and healthy people who made exercise and healthy eating a priority," she says. "They helped me to see that another life was possible for me." Carrie realized, "We all want to change the world, but the world only changes when we change ourselves."

As Fyodor Dostoevsky wrote, and Carrie knows this firsthand, "A new philosophy, a way of life, is not given for nothing. . . . It is only acquired with much patience and great effort." Carrie put in the effort, and along the way she found friends who made the effort that much easier.

In fact, research by a Southern Methodist University psychologist Jasper Smits and his colleague, Michael Otto, from Boston University, suggests that the medical profession ought to prescribe exercise more often as an effective remedy against depression and anxiety disorders.

And the anecdotal evidence mounts. . . .

Sarah, a self-described bike hound, also kicked depression via sports. She traded in a bad habit of drugs for a healthy addiction to rugby in her second year of college. "Rugby became my reason to live."

According to Sarah, the practices and games got her out of bed, into the sunshine, and around supportive people, which helped her battle the depression that had led her to drugs in the first place.

"Playing rugby felt incredibly natural to me," she says, though she had never played a team sport before. "I'd been too shy and too traumatized by my own family's addiction and depression issues to develop the trust and camaraderie with teammates that sports demanded."

But Sarah was open to a new way of being, and she learned to make friends and trust people again. "Playing rugby was the one time where I simply *was*." No need for drugs, no need to hold others at a distance in case they hurt her. "To this day, my closest friends are women I met in that period of my life."

HE LOVES ME, HE LOVES ME NOT

Making new friends can be an aphrodisiac, especially when the first rush of attachment grows beyond platonic friendship. Many a romance has been ignited on the road. Endorphins surge, pheromones collide, and the supercharged chemistry just *clicks*. Mostly it's great, as we'll see in a moment, but sometimes the sparks fly between the wrong people and casualties ensue. Welcome to the dark side, where we'll spend only a short time, since most of us don't need much of a reminder of it!

Michelle, the mountain biking single mother from California, wasn't always single. Her ex-husband was a triathlete and doctor. Work and training kept him out of the house more often than in, and after their second child was born, their relationship got rocky. Both avid runners, they couldn't seem to coordinate their schedules to ever train together.

"He said he didn't want to be slowed by a jogging stroller, even though I used it without any problem on the packed trails around the San Francisco Bay Area, where we ran," Michelle says. "He preferred training with his buddies, all men. And then somewhere along the line a woman joined them. He began to spend more time training with her instead of the guys. And of course they were doing the same races together. We were in marriage counseling at the time, and I just had a feeling. . . ."

By this point, they had drifted so far apart and were so at odds with each other that they began tiptoeing around the topic of separation. According to Michelle, it all came to a head one weekend when she took their two boys to visit her sister for the weekend.

 "When she asked if he wanted to pursue a relationship with his new training partner or try and salvage their marriage, he didn't hesitate in his answer."

"I came home and discovered small things amiss, like the dining room candles burned nearly to their base and romantic CDs in the player. I knew she'd been there. The tip-off came when she mistakenly sent him an email to our joint account that was pretty passionate. I'll leave it at that."

When Michelle confronted him, he admitted everything. When she asked if he wanted to pursue a relationship with his new training partner or try and salvage their marriage, he didn't hesitate in his answer. He wanted to be with *her*, the other "her."

"I felt like he'd been stolen from me by triathlons in some sense," Michelle says. "But now I realize how much happier I am."

And in a strange twist of events, she and his new wife have become friends, even sharing training tips, though not, one imagines, tips on how to woo your training partner.

"Of course, at the time I resented her darkly. Now I want to send her a thank-you note for her unwitting role in liberating me."

Other times the romantic sports triangle is less damaging, yet still hurtful.

Take my friend Emily, who along with her husband competed regularly in triathlons. The issue? Her husband had a female training partner, another mutual friend named Beth, and he had the unfortunate tendency of heaping a bit too much praise on her. One night while I was having dinner with them, we happened to be talking about Beth, and he offered this observation: "She has a perfect triathlon physique." When I heard the statement, I leaned back in my chair, fearing second-degree burns in the ensuing conflagration. Their fight came later, when I was out of the way.

For Emily, this crossed the line beyond mere compliment because it implied that her own triathlete body was somehow less perfect for the sport. "I didn't know if I was more hurt or furious," Emily told me later. "He could *try* to remember who he's married to." And I was reminded of the beautiful tri-suit tan line that showed in her backless wedding gown the month after the couple had done Ironman Lake Placid together. Emily was proud of her athleticism, and her husband's comment hit a tender spot.

A pall fell over the dinner and our gathering ended more quickly than it might have. Emily gave me a look, and I knew I'd hear more at our next workout. The triangle lasted another year, until Emily had a child and her husband changed his approach to sports.

"I couldn't stand Beth for a while there," Emily says, "it was like I had to blame her for stealing his attention, because otherwise I would have had to blame him. I know nothing happened, but it wasn't healthy for any of us."

When our workout partners are someone else's husband or boyfriend, we can sometimes get caught in a tension-filled triangle. On or off the road, a triangle is a shape with a lot of sharp points.

But triangles aren't the only shape, as they say. Okay, no one actually says that, except me, here on this page. There are nicer geometrical shapes, like the embrace of the circle that forms around us when we meet our life partners. As a matter of fact, many of the women I interviewed met their mates on the road.

How wonderful to share sports with our mate. Especially considering that research by UCLA psychologists showed that our pain thresholds go up at the mere thought of a loved one. In other words, if we are even just *thinking* of someone we love, we can tolerate more pain. In the study, a heat stimuli (i.e., ouch that

"In other words, if we are even just *thinking* of someone we love, we can tolerate more pain."

hurts) was applied to the forearms of women, who were simultaneously shown a series of pictures (including stranger's faces and, of all things, chairs), finishing with a photo of their boyfriends. The women were to report on the amount of pain they experienced. Researchers were looking for differences in the levels reported, depending on what picture was on view. The result? When looking at their boyfriend's picture, the women reported experiencing the least amount of pain. How much better is it if the person you love is actually with you during your workout? Not only do our loved ones feed our energy, inspiring us to do our best, but they're like an analgesic (goodbye Advil, hello handsome)—you feel less pain, so you work out harder. I could get addicted to love, better than painkillers any day.

Katrine, the triathlete in the advertising business, very astutely married a painkiller. She and her husband do triathlons together. In fact, to save money at their wedding they "ran away" together at the end. Instead of jumping into an expensive limousine, they donned running shoes and triathlon race belts (elasticized waist belts about an inch wide, on which you pin your race number) with signs that said "Just Married" and jogged off into the sunset, still in wedding clothes. More—their three-tier wedding cake depicted two figures engaged in each of the triathlon sports. Evidence that they had surely earned their cake, and no doubt enjoyed eating it, too.

 "'I fell in love with the first boy who could run as fast as me on the playground.'"

Still more love . . . this is what Suzan Wallace, the arts teacher and licensed sailing captain, told me, "I fell in love with the first boy who could run as fast as me on the playground." A story straight out of Greek myth—reminding me of Atalanta, who declared she would only marry the man who could beat her at a foot race, knowing none could. She was ultimately enticed into marriage by Melanion, who enlisted the assistance of Aphrodite to help him distract Atalanta from the race with delicious apples. We women are so easily distracted by apples—all to good cause, of course.

All these romantic stories make me want to say, "Me too, me too!"

Because, in fact, I *did* find my own painkiller out on the road.

It was our first run together, and the miles disappeared beneath our feet. Every breath of cold winter air wasabi-seared our nostrils. The New York skyline, softened by its cloak of darkness, was bejeweled with a thousand sequined windows. We talked nonstop, in that way that happens when you want to know everything about someone, where every word seems to confirm a connection that predates this lifetime. *You think that, too? You've done that, too?* The run flowed without pause into dinner in our running clothes, as if taking the time to go home and change into our street clothes might have been too long a separation to bear. Everything blurred into one unstoppable conversation ranging from running to "How did you find yourself in New York?" to the Canadian identity cri-

 "I knew already that I could take my heart out and put it in his hands for safekeeping."

sis, Jacques Derrida, deconstructionism, and international human rights standards (I was immersed in studies for my Masters of Law at the time). In just a few short hours I felt more comfortable, more myself, than ever before; I knew already that I could take my heart out and put it in his hands for safekeeping.

Our conversation continues to this day, as do our runs and our skis and our swims and our hikes and our kayaks and our snowshoes and, and, and. . . .

Sports were only one of the many elements that knitted us together, but sports and getting out into nature has always been one important source of our mutual and individual vitality, energy, and engagement. Sports knit us closer to our friends and partners, enriching our deep connections.

ME, MYSELF, AND I

As much as I cherish my friends and partner on the road, I also treasure the healing power of solitude, time alone with myself, when there's only me and the voices inside my head to keep me going.

Companionship, camaraderie, support . . . not all of us look for those things in our sports. Sometimes the athletic effort and the chatter of our minds are more than enough to keep us company. Like a moving meditation, the energetic physicality and the solitude may be just what we need to shake off the detritus of the day, to find psychic space to work out difficult problems, to allow our minds to open creatively, to refind center, and to simply breathe in, breathe out. A solitary workout can be an opportunity to reboot.

Justine, the sixty-plus marathoner who works in the film business, has never run with a partner. She runs alone and it's "a singular thing," just for her. In her work life, in the film business, she's very social. She organizes one of the premiere film festivals in the United States, and that involves way too many meetings, meals, and events with a high-octane, high-maintenance crowd. Running ensures she carves out time alone to decompress so that when she steps back into the kinetic social realm of work and play, she has the energy to fully engage.

But doing our sports alone offers so much more than the refreshment of solitude; the alone time can, paradoxically, also be much-needed company.

Krysia Hepatica, a newly-single mother, discovered how much cycling could fill up her life when she began riding to help the healing process during her divorce.

"My bike is a great outlet for me when I'm alone, without the kids. I no longer feel lonely. I'm outside. I'm watching the world as I cycle past. And I feel like I have a purpose, something I'm doing and somewhere I'm going."

Most of us spend so much time either with other people or plugged into some form of distraction, whether it's work or entertainment, that we can forget how heady time alone can be. As exciting as it is to make new friends, the experience of befriending our own selves can be equally dizzying. *Hi, stranger. Have we met before?*

I talk to myself when I'm alone. And I don't just mean inside my head. I mean *out loud,* as in, who is that crazy woman? Me,

"As exciting as it is to make new friends, the experience of befriending our own selves can be equally dizzying."

myself, and I have had quite vigorous discussions out on the trails together, sorting out problems, giving each other encouragement, brainstorming story ideas. I'm on with what Anne Thomas, a writer and marathoner, told me, "Running is my church." And the overhead costs are so much cheaper than organizing a whole religion.

Actually, many of the spiritual traditions in the world have traditions of solitude, from monastic retreats to vision quests. Science has confirmed the therapeutic effects of time on our own—showing that reducing the usual modern day sensory input levels can allow us to rest more deeply, physically, and emotionally; gain better access to our unconscious, and thus our creativity and problem solving abilities; as well as restore our energy, enabling us to strengthen our relationships and face daily life with more equanimity.

Tiffany Anderson, a freelance science writer, says she should know better by now to carry something to write with when she runs. "Some of my biggest epiphanies about how to distill dry scientific research into a vivid story that will engage non-science readers come when I'm running. It's like a flower just bursts into bloom in my brain, and I feel the thought almost physically as I run."

And check out her creative solution for capturing bursts of creativity. "I carry my cell phone with me when I run on the back trails, so if I have a breakthrough thought, I just text myself." Smarty-pants. I wonder if she thought of it on a trail run? I'm going to learn from her.

For Heidi, the marathoner and social worker, running is also a time to subconsciously work on issues in her life, to process thoughts, and have space and time for relaxation. Since her job requires so much giving and listening to others and helping them find equilibrium in their lives, she relishes the opportunity to just *be* that running provides. "I'm adding to *me*," she says.

And by adding to ourselves, we can add to the world.

ALL TOGETHER NOW

When we're feeling the restorative juices of solitary time flowing back through our veins, then we're much more ready to rejoin our community of mates, and get the most out of it.

When Mary Beth created the fitness community, AlaVie, in 2004, she and her cofounder's express intention was to create a "team" environment for women who wanted to be active but didn't have the time or training to just pick up and play soccer or participate in some other team sport.

"I feel very lucky to have played soccer for most of my life," she says. "It's easy for me to join a team. But for so many women who don't know how to play team sports, it's harder to stay active because they don't have the team environment to motivate them."

And that's what's at the heart of AlaVie—to provide multi-week fitness programs done team-style, in groups of women, often outdoors, focusing on the collective and individual goals of the participants. The team spirit AlaVie creates is even more effective than Mary Beth had expected.

"'What I didn't anticipate,' Mary Beth says, 'is how quickly and deeply the women in my programs would bond.'"

"What I didn't anticipate," Mary Beth says, "is how quickly and deeply the women in my programs would bond." Mary Beth discovered that she was meeting a need that was even greater than she'd imagined—the women she serves *crave* the community that AlaVie provides, and they flourish in a group of supporters with whom they share the same fitness goals.

Mary Beth is not the only one to discover this hunger for community among women. Laura, founder of the New York–based all-female triathlon organization Team Lipstick, discovered pretty quickly that she needed to factor "chat" time into her team workouts. The women she trains, who range from beginner to elite athletes, are "always talking." No wonder. Deep friendships form quickly when like-minded women come together, whether it's to train for their first triathlon or to knit a sweater.

"I worried at first that an all-women's team might get cliquey," admits Laura. To her relief, they didn't. "I think it's because there are no men in the mix to create that special competitiveness that can develop when women are vying for a man's attention." Instead, Laura finds that in every new group she coaches, the women bond together almost immediately, leaving no one behind, in a powerful example of cross-generational friendship. The women on her team go from strangers to bridesmaids in a matter of months, incorporating each other into their lives, as if they'd known each other for ages.

What Mary Beth and Laura observe on a regular basis was recently confirmed in a study out of the University of Copenhagen. The researchers looked at, among other things, the likelihood that women would stick with an active program. They studied women in running groups and women on soccer teams; and what they found was that the women who played soccer became more committed to the activity than the runners. Why? Because, the researchers report, "[with] the creation of we-stories . . . the soccer players were more committed to the activity itself, including the fun and not letting down teammates."

I like that expression, "we-stories," and that's what teams provide, even when the sport itself is individual.

I recently saw a clip from a forthcoming documentary titled, *Goals for Girls,* about girls playing soccer in the slums of Buenos Aires. I usually think of Argentina as a nation of soccer fanatics, where everyone grows up with a ball practically attached to their foot. But it turns out that only applies to boys and men. When it comes to girls, well, that's another story. Not only are the girls in the film battling poverty and lack of opportunity, they are battling sexism. Yet they find joy in the sport, in the "we-stories" they create. As one girl says, "When I'm sad and depressed, soccer cheers me up, because I'm with my friends."

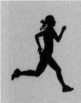 **"There's a deep sense of belonging that comes from participating in a sport, from engaging with others who share your passion. . . . "**

In addition to companionship and friendship, there's a deep sense of belonging that comes from participating in a sport, from engaging with others who share your passion, and whose attitudes and sensibilities reflect your own, in some small way.

Mushing is a distinctly solitary sport, except for the canine companionship, but one that has a deeply rooted community surrounding it nonetheless. Remember Jodi? The musher from Alaska? Well, despite her platoon of four-legged friends, socializing remains a real challenge. "I have to work on keeping relationships with people active. It is too easy to get involved with only the dogs."

Still, she has close mushing friends who understand the demands of the sport. The downside is that the women live at least a day's drive from one another, so most of their friendship is conducted online. And when they do see each other, it's to race against each other, which to an outsider might sound antithetical to friendship. But in their case the competition is not. Because the upside of their friendship is that they understand each other in profound ways that no one else can. Given the unique rigors of the sport, I can well imagine why. They belong to a special community and that creates an intense kinship.

When they *do* get together, watch out! Jodi and her three closest mushing girlfriends call themselves the "Divas," an honorific that refers to the fact that after ten days spent racing the Yukon Quest (and I think it goes without saying that there are no showers en route), they trade their well-used Michelin Man snow gear for something a little different.

"We go the whole nine yards to dress up for the finishers' banquet. We even put on pantyhose, which is completely out of place for us cabin-dwelling dog mushers." Then it's back to the dogs, and the Divas stay in touch via the ether.

When life works, we find the communities to which we belong.

"There's nothing that I am and can become that the world of martial arts won't hold," says Michelle, the founder of the Society for Martial Arts Instruction, who found her place in the male-dominated world of karate. Martial arts gave her a sense of belonging in the world in a way she'd never experienced before. When she tells the story of her early years in karate, as we've already heard, it seems improbable that it could be a place she belonged. And yet, the camaraderie and the discipline of karate spoke to Michelle.

"First it's about knowing yourself," she says. "Then it moves from self to other. We deepen the knowledge of ourselves through our relationships to others in the martial arts, by truly understanding that our biggest enemy is the one within, not our opponent on the floor."

Virginia, the sixth-degree black belt and karate teacher, says that participating in the martial arts is akin to assuming another family. "The friendships span age, gender, race, and disabilities," she says, and even transcend the competitive spirit. On the rare occasions that Virginia is beaten in a competition by another woman, rather than sulking from her loss, she hugs her competitor. "I'm proud to have such talented female competition."

Making new friends as an adult can be exhilarating.

"Clicking" with a new person and community brings its own brand of excitement, different from the absolute comfort and deep contentment of an old friendship; but then, every old friend was once a new friend.

Sam joined a local running club as a way of refilling an empty nest after her daughters were gone. "The club was similar to the bar, Cheers, where everybody knows your name," she says. "People of all shapes, sizes, careers, and ages gathered to run." Sam soon realized that the "running club" was really just a front for so much more—in addition to the running races, the club calendar was filled with football pools, weekend wine tours, biking trips, and hiking adventures. And if a club member wasn't running a particular race, they'd be there to cheer, with cups of water and Gatorade. Sam's nest got pretty full again, with a new style of family.

After all, family comes in many forms, though for most of us it starts out at home when we're young.

Tanya, the youngest of five children, started downhill skiing when she was three years old. She was initially left at the bottom of the slope to amuse herself. I know, I know—*what???*—this was back in the day (not actually so long ago), well before the time of institutionalized ski schools and hypervigilant child minding. Family members would check on her as they finished their runs. Not one to be left out of the fun, Tanya took matters into her own little hands and queued herself up for the poma lift (for the uninitiated, this is an old-fashioned ski lift comprised of a hanging vertical metal bar with an attached metal disc that fits between your legs and behind your bum, much like a rope swing). She made her way up, off, and down the mountain on her own, and then joined her family on the slopes. She never looked back.

Tanya went on to become one of the first women's freestyle skiers on the amateur circuit and admits that the social element was an enormous part of the draw. "We were always giving each other lifts to the mountain, showing off for each other. I derive my energy from people," she says. "I need the camaraderie."

These communities, particularly when it's a more formal grouping like a team, can be so much more than camaraderie though.

Linda Porter, the program director at the National Institute of Neurological Disorders and Strokes, described the "euphoria" of a good row.

"When you have a set of people who row well together, and the timing is working, and the weather is perfect, this 'thing' happens. I can't describe the feeling in words, we are pulled together, and the moment is outrageous."

When that unique "synchronicity of the universe" happens, Linda feels like she is something special in the world. "Why did I deserve this? How did I get so lucky?" The experience is so profound that it literally alters her physical appearance. The moment she walks in the door, home from the rowing workout, her sons will say, "Oh, Mom had a good one today." They can see the glow, the aura of the divinity of her experience.

Divine, yes. To be with a friend, sharing the trail . . .

On a spring Saturday, I met an intrepid friend of mine who loves to run New York City. He'll take a vague look at a map of the city and then off he goes. He has no real goals on the runs, except perhaps to run every bridge in the five boroughs and clock some miles. So here I was, joining him for one of his long urban perambulations, perched high above Hell's Gate, the watery access route to Long Island Sound. A foot away, eight lanes of high speed traffic blew past in a vortex of wind, my only protection—if you can call it that—an eight-foot-high, schoolyard-style metal fence. We were running across the Triborough Bridge, which is rarely crossed by foot but is traversed regularly by thick ribbons of motorists spooling back and forth to JFK and LaGuardia airports. At first blush the situation didn't seem all that appealing, *or* smart. But wow—what a rush to be up there, so simultaneously small and huge. Like I owned the massive city stretched out at our feet—miniaturized by distance and loft.

Not long after that, on route to the airport one day, I stared out the taxi window, looking but not seeing the hustle of the familiar world pass by. Then it struck me. I was on the Triborough again! I looked over at the empty pedestrian walkway and thought, *Jon brought me here*. I felt the *woosh* of the traffic rushing by again, and the thought made me smile to myself and then laugh out loud.

The places friends can take us. . . .

CHAPTER 8:

Tossing Our Lace Caps

"[W]hen you're swimming in the water, I know that the water doesn't know what age we are . . . age is just a number."
—Dara Torres, 41-year-old silver medalist in swimming (2008 Olympics)

T ahoe Donner, one of my favorite cross-country ski centers, often holds community races. Anyone can sign up. As a spectator at one recently, I was struck by the range of ages in the race. In the junior division, a girl of fourteen led the race, faster even than all the boys. In the adult division, women of every size, age, and ability were giving the race their all. One woman in particular wowed me. Impossible to miss in her fire engine red lycra outfit, she skate-skied powerfully through the turn near my spectator's perch, strong and lean, her snow-white hair gleaming in the sun. Late-sixties, and she finished in the top twenty. The snow obviously didn't know her age. I might also add that she was not the only woman in her age group. I don't know which side of the spectrum was more inspiring: youth and possibility, or age and possibility. I hope that young girl knows how much she is capable of. For myself, I'd like to earn some red lycra late into my sixties.

No matter how young—or less young—we are; no matter what life is throwing at us—from career pressures and new family, to disease and death—we can find our place in sports, and sports can find its place in our lives. Not only that, we will reap the rewards of its antioxidizing, de-stressing, energizing effects. Instead of feeling like the crunchy, worn-out waistband of our favorite decade-old pair of running shorts, we can be as resilient as elastic so fresh it leaves red lines on our skin. *Snap!* That's the sound effect of sports in our life. Not to mention the bonus feature—yes, I'm back on *that* hobby horse again—happiness.

WISER AND MORE MATURE, BUT NO LESS FUN

People ask seventy-five-year-old Vici DeHaan why she still gets out and does what she does, which includes, not only vigorous hikes, but also a little ultra running thrown in to boot. She says, "Because I still can." Sounds right to me. And then she adds, "I hike with a group of ladies who are also in their seventies. Young people who see us, a bunch of grandmas on the trail, are sometimes inspired to keep going so that they, too, can be hiking when they get to our age. So I guess we'll all just keep on truckin.'"

As Anne O'Hagan wrote in the *Munsey Magazine* at the turn of the century: "[A]thletics . . . have robbed old age of some of its terrors for women. . . . It is a magnificent institution which has exchanged her felt slippers for the calfskin boots of the athlete, and has delayed for fifteen or twenty years the purchase of the lace cap of her decrepitude."

Indeed—ski caps, yes; lace caps, no thanks. Let's also not forget that when O'Hagan wrote those words, she was probably referring to any woman over forty. And lest we think all that's changed now, think again. Our society still seems bent on propagating the myth that we need special attention to know "how to stay fit after forty." Sometimes when I catch a whiff of that attitude in the air, I can feel my used-to-be-a-lawyer hackles rising, and I want to enumerate the reasons it just isn't so (in the first place, with two sub-clauses). We women have not *lost* something by getting older we have *gained* strength, endurance, and psychological maturity.

As Mary, the teacher and coach, says, "The mental part of any game is usually the most important. For example, there is a lot of strategy in volleyball and you have to know your opponent. The young might have the energy and the power, but I have seen seasoned veterans beat them time and again, simply because they really 'know' how to play the game."

Psychological maturity is not just about knowing "how" to play the game, that maturity brings with it a deeper understanding of what we are truly capable of, and I don't mean the limits of our capability, I mean the *expansiveness* of our capacity.

"As an athletic woman over forty, I couldn't help but wonder if I was supposed to be slowing down."

I learned that the summer I was forty-two. As an athletic woman over forty, I couldn't help but wonder if I was supposed to be slowing down. I learned the answer without further ado. And as Mary said, I think a lot of my performance had to do with the mental part.

To start the summer off, I finished my eighth marathon fifteen minutes faster than my previous best marathon time. A month later, I competed head-to-head (or toe-to-toe, as it were) with a girl twenty-five years younger than me during a small town Fourth-of-July 5k. She was a lanky seventeen-year-old with a winged-shoe pendant hanging around her neck. She kept me honest for the first two miles, and then her speed began to flag, ceding the road to me. Then a few weeks later at my local triathlon, I was "seeded" into the younger age group, which afforded me a good swim start. For those unfamiliar with triathlons, the race sequence is always swim-bike-run. The swim start is usually done in what's called "waves," groups of racers starting two or three minutes apart. For example, men up to the age of forty might start in a wave together, then men over forty, then women up to forty, followed by women over forty. The bigger the race, the more waves there are, and the more finely sliced the categories. As you can imagine, the later the wave you start in, the more people there are swimming ahead of you. And if you are a fast swimmer, it just means more people to swim around, over, and under. Yes, it can get a little crowded in the water, so getting a good swim start is important to having your best race. I was pleased at the finish line to have earned my seeded place.

Was I physically stronger than previous years? Possibly. But that wasn't the most important factor. My *mind* was stronger. After all the noise of youth and figuring out what to do with my life, I had finally reached a place where I had time to take stock of where I was and where I was going, of what was important and what I was capable of. To my surprise, I discovered that instead of narrowing my goals and ambitions in life, I found that age was expanding them, including in athletics. I was simultaneously more determined in my pursuit of athletic goals, and less wrapped up in the outcome. The "apocalypse" just seems to come less often now that I'm older, which is good news, since it frees me up for productive things. Instead of angsting over all the perceived crises I can't change, I'm enjoying the individual moments that are happening right now.

In these pages, you've heard many women's stories of coming into their strength. And isn't strength, and the happiness that comes from it, the point? Here's another one, but it's not the last, not yet.

 "'[T]here have been times after doing something really, really hard when I feel like I could eat impossible for breakfast!'"

Jodi spent her young life as an overweight, nonathlete. She's still trying to adjust to being a forty-year-old athlete, let alone an athlete at all; even more, as a musher making her way to the top of the sport. As Jodi says, "Redefining your self-image is one of the things you do when you redefine your body or attitude or lifestyle. Of course, it isn't always easy. . . . But there have been times after doing something really, really hard when I feel like I could eat impossible for breakfast!"

Sounds delicious.

Sports play a dynamic role in our lives, changing with us as we change, meeting our ever-evolving needs. And just when we think we are getting too old for something, sports help us to think again.

Rebecca, the world champion adventure racer, is not nearly ready for retirement at the power age of forty-something, but she's already thinking about how to exit gracefully from the most competitive level of the sports she participates in. She wants to share her experiences with other women, to help them realize their dreams. The "legacy" she wants to leave isn't the list of her *own* accomplishments, but those of the women she's inspired.

What we want as we get older changes. Our relationship with sports changes. And sports change us. Not necessarily in that order, it's a lifelong cycle.

When I spoke with Sarah, who worked for a decade with the Women's Sports Foundation, she had recently returned from months of traveling around the world, an outward journey through new geography and an inward journey to consider the landscape of her possible future. But the trip didn't come without sacrifice or risk. She left a great job and a long-term relationship to take time to find her own path. She needed to pull up stakes and throw away the safety net for the trip to work, which it did, setting her on a new course toward integrating her passion for writing and film with her deep desire to give back to the world. Sports, she says, taught her to take those kinds of risks. And risk can bring reward, the reward of a transformed life. As Sarah says, "Transformation is cumulative. Every time I get myself up after a failure, it reminds me who I am and what I'm capable of."

The health benefits of sports are cumulative as well, particularly as we begin to whizz past our birthdays. . . .

THERE'S NO AGING OUT

Not that this news is a surprise, but it's always worth stating—as we age, our athletic endeavors have antiaging benefits. Really. The Harvard School of Public Health analyzed data from more than 13,000 women and found that those who were most active during middle age were more likely to be in better overall health when they were seventy or older, particularly in areas such as cognitive ability and chronic disease.

More—scientists are now confirming that exercise has an antiaging impact at the cellular level. Apparently, in our white blood cells there are things called "telomeres," which are tiny caps on the end of DNA strands. When cells divide and replicate the long DNA strands, the telomere cap is snipped, a process that is believed to protect the rest of the DNA but results in an ever-shorter telomere. At a certain point the telomeres are so short that the cell dies, or enters a sort of suspended state. The length of the telomere, then, is indicative of cellular age. To put this in context, the telomere length of a sedentary middle-aged person in the study was 40 percent shorter than a twenty-something subject. Not so for middle-aged *athletes,* whose telomeres were only a mere 10 percent shorter than runners half their age. That's a 75 percent difference. Forget about flat abs, I want to get me some long telomeres!

Still and all, I wasn't born yesterday, so I know that despite my summer of forty-two and my possibly longish telomeres, I know, too, that our capacity and strength will "change" (yes, that is a euphemism for "diminish"), as will our attitude and approach to sports. And dealing with the inevitability of those changes is part of the balancing act.

> "'[I]t wasn't the pain that made me cry, it was the thought that my body might be growing older. . . .'"

Lynn, the devotee of all mountain sports, is in her late forties. And while still strong by all standards, she says her age has an impact on her nonetheless. "As I grow older my body is giving me trouble. Last winter, on a day where we skied twenty miles in about six hours, carrying multiday packs the whole way, the pain I felt in my back brought me to tears. But it wasn't the pain that made me cry, it was the thought that my body might be growing older and might not let me go so far into the backcountry anymore."

Change is often bittersweet. Yet if we hang on to what once *was,* how much less happy we will be than if we revel in the possibilities of what *can be.* "When my body asks me to slow down," Lynn says, "I can think of a hundred other things I'd like to be doing—spending time with my niece, painting a wall in my condo, baking, reading, hanging with friends who don't participate in my mountain adventures. Patience . . . "

Earlier I mentioned beating a few younger runners. And while those races were self-affirming (I'm not done yet!), my favorite "youngster" to beat is myself.

While I was studying for my undergraduate degree at McGill University in Montreal, I had a passing relationship with the concept of running. Every once in a while I would put on sweats (yes, those big bulky gray cotton pantaloons) and try to run up Mont Royal, the bump in the middle of Montreal from which the city got its name. The mountain (such as it is) is actually a lovely run up a gently graded dirt road that winds around the mountain a few times, until the path reaches the lookout at the top. Back then I couldn't make the top. Actually, I could barely *start*. Most days I hardly made it the few blocks to the base of the running path before I was walking. A couple of years ago, I had occasion to be in Montreal. Every morning, I woke early and ran up that mountain. And what charged me up most, aside from the pretty bridle path enclosed in an avenue of trees, was the thought of myself at eighteen years old, huffing and puffing, stopping and walking, wondering how anyone ever ran to the top, then going back to my dorm for a cigarette (and yes, that was the most important butt I've ever kicked). Like Lynn, I know that I won't always be able to beat the younger versions of myself, so I'm enjoying the moments now and looking forward to finding new challenges the younger me never even dreamed of.

Besides, I may have some time yet, if Ruth Rothfarb, Jenny Wood-Allen, or Zofia Turosa are any indication of what the future holds. At eighty-six and ninety, respectively, Ruth and Jenny both finished the Boston Marathon in recent years. As for seventy-one-year-old Zofia, in 2009 *she* finished in 4:19. According to the fancy age-grading tables developed by the United States Track and Field Association, Zofia's time converts to a 2:42 marathon for an equivalent woman in her so-called "prime." In fact, a little over twenty years ago, Zofia ran her first Boston Marathon in just under three hours. Zofia has eschewed the lap pool, usually considered the most suitable venue for women her age, and instead runs 60 miles a week.

Yes, Zofia's pace has changed, but so, no doubt, have her expectations.

Like Zofia, sixty-something Kathrine Switzer, the first woman to run the Boston Marathon legally (if not welcomely) in 1967, says she has changed her relationship with running more than once over the years. When she hit menopause, she says it was the first time her body felt completely outside her control. The only time she felt good was when she was running.

"I felt like I still had my magic," she says.

Nowadays, the relationship has morphed even more. After thirty-five marathons, she finds that a regular road marathon no longer holds allure for her. Instead, she is seeking new challenges, like the Motatapu. This 49-kilometer endurance run (that's 7k longer than a marathon, for the record) climbs over a range of mountains in New Zealand, on protected land that is only open to the public once a year, and only for the race.

Motatapu is Kathrine's way of "slowing down," running on theoretically gentler terrain than the roads, even if the race is long and arduous. As she wrote post-race, "Let me say, I was a bit out of my mind to choose one of the hardest endurance races in New Zealand: through the mountainous high country, carrying a pack, twenty-eight river crossings, all off-road with astonishing descents as well as ascents. I finished in five hours, thirty-eight minutes; average time for women over fifty is over six hours, so I am exceedingly pleased. Mostly to know an old body can gear up again and embrace adventure."

Embrace adventure, yes, that's really what life is all about. And since the spirit of adventure happens first in our minds, there's no aging out.

Donna, who recently retired from a career in human resources is an expert caver and climber and has traveled the world in search of the best caves and mountains to explore. "My sports have created an opportunity to live a unique, gypsy lifestyle," she says. And she seems to be one of those rare people who always

"[S]ince the spirit of adventure happens first in our minds, there's no aging out."

understood the possibilities life offered, something she says she knew at a young age. "I wasn't destined for an ordinary life. I didn't want to look back and say, 'I wish I would have. . . .'" Now close to sixty years old, she has fulfilled her dreams and ambitions, but that hasn't stopped her from forging new challenges, new goals.

"My husband and I decided to retire early, so for the last three years we have been in living in an RV and traveling around the Western United States, mainly climbing, but also skiing during the winter. Now that we can engage in sports all the time, we set ambitious goals and enjoy the journey to achieving them all the more. I feel like my life has come full circle. When I was younger, I left my job to climb, and traveled around in a beat up old car. Now that I am older, I left my job to climb and travel around, but at least in a much better vehicle, and with the love of my life. Life is good."

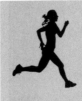

> **"One thing is certain—and I don't mean death or taxes. It's *change*."**

One thing is certain—and I don't mean death or taxes. It's *change*. In our bodies, our attitudes, our goals, and abilities. By running like a girl into that future, we can welcome the new and the different with open arms. Fast has its time. Slow has its time.

RUN LIKE A MOTHER

For many women, one of the "slow times" (at least athletically) is pregnancy, followed by the harried early years of motherhood, in which finding time to shower is a gift, never mind finding time for sports.

And yet motherhood, as so many women have proven, need not be the end of sports, but more of an alteration, a reimagining of how sports fit in.

And it can start right from the beginning, when "Z" (for zygote), as we called my youngest brother in-utero, first announces its presence. Yet some doctors, particularly old-school types, still discourage women from exercising during pregnancy, believing that it's detrimental to a woman and her fetus. *Hmmm.* A little red flag might be raised here, yes? If the scaremongers are to be believed, how did we make it this far in our evolution as a species? Forget history. Even now, outside of what we think of as the developed world, women hardly confine themselves to bed for the duration, and there is no shortage of children in those regions (other short-ages, of course, but those would likely be made worse if women were encouraged to "slow down").

But no need to rely on me (and don't trust my stock tips either). A recent report published in the *Journal of the American Academy of Orthopedic Surgeons* recommended that physicians should actually *prescribe* moderate levels of exercise to their pregnant patients, even if they had never exercised before. Why? Well, aside from the obvious—that it strengthens musculoskeletal and physiologic health—it also significantly reduces just about all the ailments typically associated with pregnancy: back pain, high blood pressure, swelling, muscle pain, and postpartum depression. And of course, what's good for the goose is good for the gosling (okay, that's not quite how the saying goes). . . .

And once our babies are born? Well I'll let others more expert on the topic speak to that.

 "'We need to be healthy in mind, body, and spirit if we are to be the best mothers we can be.'"

As Lisa, a literary agent, marathon runner, and mother of two, says, "We need to be healthy in mind, body, and spirit if we are to be the best mothers we can be."

With a demanding job and two boys at home, Trisha, the vice-president at a wealth management firm, believes that it's a constant dance to find the "logistical balance versus the emotional balance" of fitting running into her life. Though sports will never be the center of her existence, when she finds the time to exercise, Trisha feels more in control of her physical presence and more in tune with everything else in her life—family, work, and friends. On the flip side, when her workouts slip by the wayside, Trisha is more likely to feel that things are spiraling out of control in the rest of her life, which isn't good for anyone.

We make others happy when we are happy ourselves.

For these women, making time for their sports is akin to "putting their oxygen mask on first." Becky, the long distance swimmer and small business owner, says that when her eight-and-a-half-year-old son sees her, one of the first things he asks is, "Are you sweaty?" Not because he's grossed out by her sweat, on the contrary, he's asking because he knows that when she's sweaty, she's also happy.

The happiness, the calm, and, yes, the extra energy of being healthy, all pay dividends to our families and careers. We build our personal happiness on two pillars, the public pillar of our careers, work, and education and the private pillar of our relationships with family and friends. Finding our own right balance of energy between the two pillars is the challenge of life, a challenge where sports have proven helpful at every age and stage.

Not to mention the fact that mothers set a great example for their children when they participate.

Rebecca, a runner and advertising copywriter, came to running through her job writing copy for Garmin, the company that makes GPS-enabled super-watches for athletes. For her first marathon, she set herself the goal of qualifying for Boston (the Boston marathon requires certain minimum finish times from another marathon, depending on your gender and age). As she came into the last stretch, Rebecca's children were at the finish line, waiting for their mother to cross and qualify. But she missed the qualifying time by a mere ninety seconds, a tiny amount in a 26.2 mile race, and surely incredibly frustrating. But Rebecca knew that her daughters were watching, so she transformed the moment.

"'They knew mom had a specific goal and had worked very hard to achieve it. But when the goal wasn't met, mom didn't pack up her gear and find a new sport.'"

"I realized what an amazing lesson this would be for my kids," she says. "They knew mom had a specific goal and had worked very hard to achieve it. But when the goal wasn't met, mom didn't pack up her gear and find a new sport." Instead, Rebecca figured out where her next marathon would be.

Like anything else in life—going away to university, a new job, a new relationship—when you have children you adjust to accommodate the changes.

When Laural, the adventure mentor, first met her husband, she was into long bike tours and he was a cycle and triathlon racer. They each tried a bit of the other's, and then "wisely," as Laural says, bought a tandem for their honeymoon to eliminate intramarital competition. When they added kids to the mix, she says it was crucial for them to figure out how to add kids to the bicycling. They tried putting their infant son in his car seat, secured into a bike trailer. Later they learned that it was not recommended to ride with children under a year old. *Oops.* They've since graduated to actual bicycle-mounted child seats and special attachments to allow the kids to be the "stoker" on a tandem (that's the person in the back). Since then, Laural and her family have gone on family bicycling trips around the world, including six weeks on the Pacific Coast of the United States and a month in Europe.

More is possible than we often think.

STANDING UP THE EIGHTH TIME

Motherhood is just one of the many life changes the universe bestows upon us. Others less predictable and certainly less rewarding may throw a wrench in our lives. Disease, divorce, death of someone cherished—these life changes can debilitate us, inside and out. And you've probably already figured out by now that sports can help us through this, too. As the old saying goes, "Fall down seven times, stand up eight."

When she was twelve years old, Samantha Redford, now a massage therapist in her early-twenties, was making divinity candy in the microwave. Unbeknownst to her, the bottom of the plastic bowl had burned through. When she took the bowl out of the microwave, the boiling sugar splashed on to her bare legs and feet. At the critical age when a girl's self-consciousness begins to peak, Samantha had the added burden of coping with severe burn scars on her legs. For several years she wore nothing but pants. But then sports called, specifically cross-country running. To run though, she needed to wear shorts. And to wear shorts, she had to overcome her embarrassment about her legs.

She did. Not only that, by virtue of the confidence she earned hurtling through the woods, she was able to turn the scars into battle wounds, into a story, into an aspect of "cool" on her high school running team. It's not that she never thinks about them anymore. Rather, she has come to peace with the scars. The pleasure she gets out of sports more than balances out any residual self-consciousness she feels about the permanent record left on her legs.

Regina Daly's body also has a permanent record of her own fight with an aggressive disease. In October 2005, Regina ran her first marathon. Two months later she woke up in the ICU of a Denver hospital, where she'd undergone the first of many surgeries to arrest the necrotizing fasciitis (NF) she had mysteriously contracted. NF is more commonly known as flesh-eating bacteria; and the

"On her first run, she didn't even bother changing into running clothes."

disease is as terrible as it sounds. To replace the missing skin on her chest, Regina had large swaths of skin removed from her armpit, neck, and chest, and skin grafts taken from the top of her thighs. It required multiple surgeries. She got out of the hospital the first week of January 2006 and went back to work February 1. She began running again in early March. She had a goal, to run the Bolder Boulder 10k, a race she'd done every year, except the year she was pregnant.

On her first run, she didn't even bother changing into running clothes. She just put on her running shoes and plodded out the door. She ran for ten minutes, but, as she says, "it was enough to get a little sweaty and start breathing hard. I was so happy when I finished that I almost started crying." Even better, she did the 10k, and later that summer she did a four-hundred-plus-mile, six-day bike tour in Colorado. Her doctors were amazed, to say the least. In October of that year, only ten months after leaving the hospital, she did the Marine Corps Marathon and finished thirty minutes faster than she had two years earlier in Chicago. Take that NF!

Sports reinforce and remind us that life is constantly moving in different directions, often all at the same time, and we can accept and adapt to the constant change without feeling defeated. After all, as George Eliot wrote in *Janet's Repentance,* "Any coward can fight a battle he's sure of winning; but give me the man who has the pluck to fight when he's sure of losing. That's my way, sir; and there are many victories worse than a defeat."

For Justine, the marathoner in the film business in her early sixties, it was a setback that got her out on the road in the first place. Four weeks before her fiftieth birthday her husband of twenty years walked out on her. "As if I'd been a one-night stand in a bar," she says.

Taking up running, particularly long distances, helped her recover. She was suddenly single and the mother of a young daughter, but she was also an athlete, and that made all the difference. Running gave her something to focus on. She didn't have much time or energy to feel sorry for herself anymore. Getting out on the road was, as Justine put it, "An intervention in that feeling of waking up alone."

But then, as running does, the pursuit took on a life of its own.

When she hit a solid hour on the treadmill, she thought, "I can run a marathon." She was right, though achieving that goal took a bit of time to execute—injuries sidelined her for the first two possible marathons. Still, Justine fought for her marathon, especially when those around her told her she needed to "stop pursuing this insane dream," and even when she was shaking from exhaustion in the shower after her first thirteen-mile run. At work and at home, among colleagues and friends, everyone said, "It's too late." An insightful orthopedist told her, "You'll figure out how to do it." And she did, running her first marathon at fifty-five years old. She's still going strong.

And Justine didn't even have Michelle, who founded Awesome Adventure Women when she herself got divorced. Her goal: to provide opportunities for women to engage with other like-minded women in outdoor activities and sports they'd always wanted to try but didn't because of the intimidation factor, circumstance, or because they simply had no one to do it with and were too uncomfortable to do it alone. From rock climbing and kayaking to wine tasting and archery, the activities Michelle hooks other women up with are as varied as the women she serves, and she provides it with a heavy dose of encouragement. Don't we all need that, at least some of the time? Sports helped Michelle through her divorce, and now she's giving back, helping other women find new sources of happiness.

For Paula, a nurse practitioner, it was her kayak that got her through some hard times. "Big Blue," as she called it, was a "free" kayak, acquired on a whim through a credit card reward's program. The bright blue two-person kayak caught her eye and she imagined skimming across a northern Wisconsin lake with her husband, even though neither had kayaked before. When the boat arrived, the two of them would stare at it out the window as they drank their morning coffee. The boat began to grow on them. Maybe they'd use it after all. And then quite out of nowhere, Paula's husband developed ALS, commonly known as Lou Gehrig's disease. Big Blue was stored and forgotten. And a year and a half later, Paula found herself a widow, sleepless, "roaming my house in search of a new life."

A few days later, without quite intending to, Paula was researching kayaking. She found lessons offered fifteen minutes from her house. The first day, the kayak instructor asked everyone why they had signed up. People said the expected—trips coming up and such. Almost everyone was part of a couple, planning a future adventure.

 "'Suddenly I blurt out, "my husband died two weeks ago. I bought a tandem kayak for us, but we never got to use it."'"

"Suddenly I blurt out, 'my husband died two weeks ago. I bought a tandem kayak for us, but we never got to use it. So I have no experience.'" There was a long silence. No one responded. Paula was embarrassed for having cast a pall on the class.

A man who had lost his wife to cancer approached Paula later in the day and congratulated her on her courage.

Seven years on, Paula has taken other kayak lessons, bought a "sleek and sultry single kayak," and has generally spent far more than she thought was possible on the sport. She's moved cities, changed careers, found new kayaking buddies, and, yes, even a new husband, who has his own single kayak. For seven years, Big Blue followed Paula around, from rafter to rafter, as she built her new life. But the boat never touched water. Paula finally placed an ad: "For sale, Big Blue." Only days later, Paula helped a family with four young boys strap the kayak on to the roof of their car, bidding her longtime fellow traveler goodbye.

As life weaves around us, sports find new places to fit, healing us, keeping us company, inspiring us, reminding us of the extraordinary.

Lois, the flight attendant who's in her early sixties, didn't realize until recently how much of a "good friend at her side" sports had been throughout her life. When she was young she enjoyed sports, but she let athletics fall by the wayside when the "cool" girls told her they'd like her more if she gave up sports. College in the sixties was all about drugs, and she spiraled downward until landing in rehab in her late thirties. Shortly before rehab, when she lived in Berlin, she remembers running at 7:00 AM after chasing a Xanax with beer. Her sister nursed her back to health in Florida, where she took up aerobics for a time. They made her feel normal for a couple of hours afterward. But slowly, she felt normal for longer periods of time.

"Sports are just a metaphor for life," Lois says, "a beginning, peaks and valleys, and an end." And by all accounts, she's far from

 "She wondered to herself, 'Can I still do that handstand off the side of the pool?' And she did."

the end. When her niece was visiting recently with her newborn, she was so inspired by their exuberant youthfulness that she wondered to herself, "Can I still do that handstand off the side of the pool?" And she did.

WE'RE NEVER TOO OLD TO BEGIN

Cooler than almost anything else about sports is that they're equal opportunity endeavors. Sports don't discriminate—against appearance, gender, size, or age. We can start any time, from age five to ninety-five. Being active has no age limit. Our sports have infinite patience—they wait for us, and when we're ready, they won't look meaningfully at their watch and complain that we took too long. And since we're all aging anyway, why not have fun with it and throw in some sports. As Dan Millman said in *Body Mind Mastery: Training for Sport and Life*, "If you're going 'over the hill' anyway, bring a kite!"

More than a kite, I'd actually call sports more of a "glider," something that eases us so much more gently into our next birthday and the one after that, and so on. At the risk of sounding like a broken record, study after study on exercise and aging shows a direct link to longevity and improved health, both mental and physical. Exercise staves off everything from Alzheimer's and Parkinson's disease to diabetes and high blood pressure. Exercise rejuvenates worn and damaged muscle tissue in healthy seniors and stimulates brain growth, preventing dementia and stroke. And the ailments that can plague us after fifty—including arthritis and achy joints— are improved from the types of exercise (like running, tennis, and cycling) that were once believed to *exacerbate* the debilitating vagaries of aging. So many studies . . . I'll mention just this one.

Beginning in 1984, researchers from Stanford University's School of Medicine began tracking five hundred older runners and compared them to their sedentary counterparts. Many scientists and physicians believed (probably still believe despite evidence to the contrary) that vigorous exercise does more harm than good when we're older, believing (for example) running would lead to floods of orthopedic injuries. The Stanford researchers thought differently. They believed regular exercise would extend high-quality, disability-free life. They were right. More than twenty years later, the runners they studied, many in their eighties, have far fewer disabilities than their nonactive counterparts, they enjoy a longer span of an active life, and are half as likely as nonrunners to die early deaths. *Half* as likely? Are you kidding me? I'm in! Red lycra, anyone?

"Here's a fun fact: our muscles, no matter how long we've neglected them, no matter if we're eighty, still have the capacity to be strengthened."

Here's a fun fact: our muscles, no matter how long we've neglected them, no matter if we're eighty, still have the capacity to be strengthened. Studies have shown that when frail sedentary women in their seventies, eighties, and nineties are put on a strength-training regimen, they experience incredible results. Better still, that muscle is good protection around our thinning bones, something we can't change as we get older.

"Muscle is gracious. It does not hold grudges. Even an elderly woman who never learned to do cartwheels or bothered to join a fitness club in early adulthood can, in her oxidized age, become a mighty virago," says Natalie Angier, in *Woman: An Intimate Geography.*

Louise, a writer who works out regularly at the gym, embraces that sentiment. "In this, the year of my seventieth birthday, I went snorkeling for the first time. An almost passive activity, I admit. But just being in a rocking ocean, maneuvering about to watch life I had never seen before, made me love my body more."

Never too late.

Linda, the program director at the National Institute of Neurological Disorders and Strokes, marathoner and rower, took up rowing in her late forties after watching her son row in high school. Actually, the rowing bug had been inside her since her youth. Growing up, her cousin was a national champion rower, but because sports were so little available to girls at the time, it didn't even occur to Linda that she could row if she wanted.

Fast forward several decades later. When the father of one of her son's teammates mentioned a "learn to row" program, she signed up immediately. Linda now dominates the master's rowing scene in Washington, D.C. She was even named "Most Valuable Player" (MVP) of her team. Not only that, at fifty-four, she rows in the forty-plus boats, not the fifty-plus boats, because she's stronger than most of the women in their forties. Actually, the influence of her strength is even cooler. Forty-plus boats are established by "averaging" the age of the four or eight rowers in the boat. As long as that average is in the forties, they're golden. That means that when Linda is pulled into a forty-plus boat, she not only adds power, she enables the boat to add in a strong woman in her thirties (if there aren't enough in their forties), because their two ages average out. A twofer. No wonder she's so valuable.

> **"All our sports will ever say is, 'Long time no see, cool to have you back. Let's play.'"**

Don't think you can't, just because you've never, no matter how old you are. And more—don't think you can't again, just because you gave up a much-loved sport in the past. Sports are not an exclusive event with no re-entry once you've left. Nope. There's no velvet rope and snooty guard keeping us out if we try to come back a second time. All our sports will ever say is, "Long time no see, cool to have you back. Let's play."

Karen, the attorney and marathoner, ran when she was young. Taller than most of the boys and all of the girls in her class, she excelled. "When I was young, I ran like the wind; I thought I had a star on my forehead." Full of confidence, she hit her teens and all of a sudden in grade 7, boys and girls were separated out for sports. This was before Title IX and that meant girls' sports were essentially ignored. The other girls thought Karen was rude and aggressive, not like a girl ought to be at all. So for Karen, sports fell away from her life for a long time. She lived vicariously through her daughter's sports. "It would make me cry to see my daughter run, remembering middle school and how I felt when I ran." Then, at fifty-one years old, she did her first marathon. "I've never seen a picture of myself so happy as when I finished that marathon."

Karen got back that star on her forehead.

Geeta, the senior executive at an education testing and curriculum development company, keeps coming back to running, which didn't hook her until college. "I was one of those theater and music geeks in high school," she says. Yet she and running have had some challenging times in their relationship. For several years she has been trying to get pregnant. Some doctors have advised her to cut back on her running. "I feel as if this activity, which has always given me so much peace, is suddenly my enemy," she says. Still, she has never completely abandoned the sport, coming back to running for solace after each unsuccessful round of in vitro fertilization. With or without a baby jogger, running will always be there for her when she needs it.

Lucky for us, our sports don't hold grudges in our absence.

But absence itself can be hard on us. It's not always easy to get back into the swing of things, let alone get into the swing of things for the first time. Being a beginner, particularly when we're at an age where we find "beginner status" to be alien and yes, even uncomfortable.

 "Just as she was getting frustrated, a woman on snowshoes asked if she was training with her high school ski team."

At a cross-country ski clinic, Kristen, the fly fishing manufacturer's representative, said, "I feel like a baby chick, being herded around and asked to do balance drills." Which, she says, often ended up with her falling over sideways in front of an audience of other skiers who stopped to watch the clinic.

"I'm forty-five, this is embarrassing," she said.

But then, just as she was getting frustrated, a woman on snowshoes asked if she was training with her high school ski team. With its apparent power to strip away the years, Oil of Olay should consider teaming up with ski clinics.

Donna had a similar feeling to Kristen's. The ceramic artist and black belt took up karate when she was in her early forties. Initially, there was an uncomfortable adjustment to being a beginner again. The first time she was tested, she thought to herself, "But I'm in my forties, who are these people to be testing me."

We reach a certain age and we feel we ought to have "arrived," whatever that means. But we'll never arrive. There's nowhere to arrive at, except death. So Donna accepted her beginner status.

At first, Donna would be worn out within the first half hour of class and have to sit down and take a break. Now, eight years later, she is, as her sensei Michelle says, "light years ahead of the person she used to be."

Other tests held other challenges along the way. Early on, Donna was voted least likely to ever get a black belt among her peers. She hated to fight, and in the particular lineage of karate she practices, full-contact fighting is an absolute requirement. In fact, fighting *is* the black belt test. So to get her black belt, Donna had to fight. And she did. She still doesn't much like fighting. But she will when necessary. Least likely to get her black belt? Apparently not.

I know that feeling too, of being a beginner long after I think that due date ought to have expired.

I recently did the second short-course cross-country ski race I'd ever done in my life. I wasn't even planning to do the race at all. I went as a spectator. But when I got there, I discovered that only one other woman was signed up, and it was fifteen minutes to race time. The race director showed me the free hats to be won, and I signed up. At the thought of "free stuff" I forgot my fear of being a beginner. But if I had stopped to consider the economics, I probably could have bought the hat for little more than the race registration fee.

I went outside to put my skis on. There was a woman in her early twenties dressed in race-ready lycra, her warm-up jacket covered with sponsors and the Norwegian flag. In a Scandinavian accent she asked me where the start was. Once I'd answered, she skied off toward the start at a ferocious pace, with perfect form. "Direct from Oslo, where they are born with skis on," my partner said, laughing. "Your competition." Indeed.

As a woman, I'm proud to say that my Scandinavian competition beat all the men. I came in a distant second among the women (okay among all six of us who raced, since a few signed up after me). The race was refreshing and low stress. I was out there to feel what it was like to go as hard as I could for the 5k distance. I learned where I needed to improve my technique to go faster. The race fired up my desire to improve, not so I could race faster, just to improve for its own sake. Because the feeling of getting better and doing something well feels like an accomplishment, each increment of skill, *empowering*.

I didn't win a free hat, but that lace cap of decrepitude?—it will have disintegrated to dust by the time I'm ready for it.

NOW IS A GOOD TIME

Are you still here with me, reading this book? Or have you taken off on some adventure, leaving this book upended on the couch, spine cracked open to these last pages, the cat gazing around, disconcerted by your sudden absence.

I know how you feel. Let's *go*.

As Kristen Ulmer, an extreme skier and spiritual teacher said in *Spiritual Adventures in the Snow*, "I don't believe when we are birthed that we are actually *born*. It is just an invitation to be born. And if we choose to go on that journey, it is there for the taking."

 "The 'use by' date isn't marked on our packaging, but the expiration is there nonetheless."

There for the taking, yes, but only for so long. After all, these treasured bodies of ours, these bodies that take us on adventures, these bodies we nourish and cherish, are only on loan to us for this lifetime. The "use by" date isn't marked on our packaging, but the expiration is there nonetheless.

Pamela Andrews, who I met at a meditation session, spent a lot of time with her mother in the last months before her mother's death. At one point, about a week before she died, Pamela's mother said, "I can feel it. I can feel that I'm starting to leave my body."

"My mother's death reminded me of how temporary our bodies ultimately are."

Temporary, fleeting, finite—while we cannot become so attached to our bodies that we can't psychologically sustain the setbacks of injuries or illness, the passing ownership is all the more reason to remember every day how precious our bodies are. How lucky we are to have bodies that will run through the blinding snow, as I did the morning before I met Pamela, or swim across a lake, or ski down a mountain, or stand in tree pose.

Brett, the former professional ski cross racer, who was fortunate enough to get away with her life in a devastating skiing accident, says, "I feel as though I've already escaped paralysis and/or death once, and I can't take that chance ever again."

Does that mean she's stopped skiing? Not at all. She shocked everyone with her eagerness to get "back on the horse." She's sworn off competing, but not off sports, not by a long shot—skiing, mountain biking, road biking, and rodeo (in this case, getting on a *real* horse) are a small sample of what she's getting up to. I would guess that Brett knows better than many of us what it's like to feel death nipping at her heels, and she's choosing to keep living to the fullest.

As Pascal Mercier wrote so beautifully, and mercilessly, in *Night Train to Lisbon*, "Who could in all seriousness want to be immortal? Who would like to live for all eternity? How boring and stale it must be to know that what happens today, this month, this year, doesn't matter: endless more days, months, years will come. . . . It is death that gives the moment its beauty."

Allison, a writer who counts her life rich with activities ranging from running to kayaking, says, "Life is the sum total of your experiences and I'm trying to collect as many as possible." Allison

"'Life is the sum total of your experiences and I'm trying to collect as many as possible.'"

took up stand-up paddle boarding just before her fortieth birthday. On a trip with college friends, she and one girlfriend spent the day in the ocean, "laughing, falling down, standing up, and having a blast," while their other friends sat on the beach moaning about the state of their lives.

I know which sounds better to me. As much as moaning can seem strangely appealing at times, laughing has a ring to it, don't you think?

And as Karen, the attorney and marathoner, says, "If I had six weeks to live I would want to spend the time outside, doing some kind of activity, feeling physically alive."

Being alive is what it's all about, isn't it? We can die before we die, by disengaging from our present, or we can live until the very last drop. *Now* is a good time.

Here is the place where I might have written, "The End." As if such a thing exists, as if we aren't all beginning, again and again, because that's what living is all about, and what sports demonstrate to us so often. So instead I want to write, "The Beginning."

The beginning of our lives is now. This moment. What we were yesterday is not immutable. What we are today can be expanded upon. There is so much we are capable of. We will never know the half of it, but it's worth the attempt. By seeking and finding happiness with deepest intention, we show others the fullness of possibility in life.

Inside each one of us is a person even grander than we have ever imagined.

Be that person.

Be happy.

Running in the summer, I find myself on a trail dropping down into the Sierra Nevada's Euer Valley, one that I cross-country ski in the winter. I've no agenda, no race I'm training for, and there is no purpose beyond pleasure. The trail is like an old familiar friend, but new. What last I saw as a winter wonderland, sparkling snow trees and an undulating desert of white, is now green and gold, the mountain tops purple-gray, the smell of pine and the sweet-sharp citrusy scent of something else I can't yet identify, though I've plunged my nose into any number of the scrubby bushes. I half expect a cowboy to appear and tip his hat to me graciously before continuing on his way.

The seasons change and come again and again, reminding me that time is passing. The world is created of infinite variety that was here before me and will remain long after I'm gone. Breathing in the beautiful world through my pores as I'm borne along by my two strong legs somehow makes the finiteness of my existence more manageable. I can only take one step at a time, whether I'm running or living.

Today is a good day.

This is my life and it's happening now.

Notes

CHAPTER 1: DO YOU RUN LIKE A GIRL?

Carlson, Susan A., et al. "Physical Education and Academic Achievement in Elementary School: Data from the Early Childhood Longitudinal Study." *American Journal of Public Health* (February 2008).

Lamott, Annie. *Bird by Bird: Some Instructions on Writing and Life.* New York: Pantheon Books, 1994.

Sandoz, Joli, and Joby Winans (editors). *Whatever It Takes: Women on Women's Sport.* New York: Farrar Straus & Giroux, 1999.

Stevenson, Betsey. "Beyond the Classroom: Using Title IX to Measure the Return to High School Sports." *The Review of Economics and Statistics 92, no. 2 (May 2010): 284–301*

Whitney Johnson, "Can 'Nice Girls' Negotiate?" Harvard Business Review Blog. http://blogs.hbr.org/cs/.

CHAPTER 2: DISCOVERING OUR MAGIC SHOES

Al Huang, Chungliang, and Jerry Lynch. *Thinking Body, Dancing Mind: Taosports for Extraordinary Performance in Athletics, Business, and Life*. New York: Bantam Books, 1992.

Cashmore, Ellis. *Sport and Exercise Psychology: The Key Concepts*. New York: Routledge, 2008.

Friedman, Sally. *Swimming the Channel: A Widow's Journey to Life*. New York: Farrar Straus & Giroux, 1996.

Gyatso, Geshe Kelsang. *Transform Your Life: A Blissful Journey*. New York: Tharpa Publications, 2007.

Martin, April. "Dreams on Ice." In *Whatever It Takes: Women on Women's Sport*, edited by Joli Sandoz and Joby Winans, 152–155. New York: Farrar, Straus & Giroux, 1999.

Millman, Dan. *Body Mind Mastery: Training for Sport and Life*. Novato, California: New World Library, 1999.

Ratey, John. *Spark: The Revolutionary New Science of Exercise and the Brain*. Boston: Little, Brown and Company, 2008.

CHAPTER 3: RISING TO THE (ALMOST) DAILY CHALLENGE

Campbell, Joseph, and Bill Moyers. "Joseph Campbell and the Power of Myth." Mystic Fire Video, 1988.

Gonzales, Laurence. *Deep Survival: Who Lives, Who Dies, and Why*. New York: W. W. Norton & Company, 2003.

Kraftsow, Gary. *Yoga for Transformation: Ancient Teachings and Practices for Healing the Body, Mind, and Heart.* Penguin Group (USA), 2002.

Lamott, Annie. Ibid.

Tolle, Eckhart. *The Power of Now: A Guide to Spiritual Enlightenment.* Novato, California: New World Library, 1999.

CHAPTER 4: THE GOLDILOCKS PRINCIPLE

Arnstein, Paul, Michelle Vidal, Carol Wells-Federman, Betty Morgan, and Margaret Caudill. "From chronic pain patient to peer: Benefits and risks of volunteering." *Pain Management Nursing* 3, no. 3 (2002): 94–103

http://spinningleese.blogspot.com/

Ironson, Gail H., et al. "Personality and HIV Disease Progression: Role of NEO-PI-R Openness, Extraversion, and Profiles of Engagement." *Psychosomatic Medicine: Journal of Biobehavioral Medicine* 70 (2008): 245–253.

Oman, Doug, Carle E. Thoresen, and Kay Mcmahon. "Volunteerism and Mortality among the Community-dwelling Elderly." *The Journal of Health Psychology* 4, no. 3 (1999): 301–316.

Shannon, Lisa. *A Thousand Sisters: My Journey into the Worst Place on Earth to Be a Woman.* Berkeley: Seal Press, 2010.

www.prettytough.com

CHAPTER 5: FIT IS THE NEW THIN

Allen, Mark, Tyler Owens, and Diane Spangler. "An fMRI study of self-reflection about body image: Sex differences." *Personality and Individual Differences* 48, no. 7 (2010): 849–854.

Angier, Natalie. *Woman: An Intimate Geography*. Boston: Houghton Mifflin Harcourt, 1999.

Cashmore, Ellis. Ibid.

Focht, Brian, Thomas Raedeke, and Donna Scales. "Social environmental factors and psychological responses to acute exercise for socially physique anxious females." *Psychology of Sport and Exercise* 8 (2007): 463–476.

Grabe, Shelly, Janet Hyde, and L. Monique Ward. "The role of the media in body image concerns among women: a meta-analysis of experimental and correlational studies." *Psychological Bulletin* 134, no. 3 (2008): 460–476.

Hoch, Anne Z., et al. "Prevalence of the Female Athlete Triad/ Tetrad in Professional Ballet Dancers." *Medicine & Science in Sports & Exercise* 41, no. 5 (2009): 524.

http://spinningleese.blogspot.com/

Lelwica, Michelle M. *The Religion of Thinness: Satisfying the Spiritual Hungers Behind Women's Obsession with Food and Weight*. Carlsbad, California: Gurze Books, 2009.

Speck, R. M., et al. "Changes in the Body Image and Relationship scale following a one-year strength training trial for breast cancer survivors with or at risk for lymphedema." *Breast Cancer Research and Treatment*, 121, no. 2 (2009): 421–430.

Women's Sports Foundation. "Her Life Depends On It II: Sport, Physical Activity, and the Health and Well-Being of American Girls and Women," 2009. www.womenssportsfoundation.org.

CHAPTER 6: CHICKING THE BOYS

Angier, Natalie. Ibid.

Fowers, Alyssa, and Blaine Fowers. "Social Dominance and Sexual Self-Schema as Moderators of Sexist Reactions to Female Subtypes." *Sex Roles* 62 (2009): 468–480.

Gneezy, Uri, John List, and Kenneth Leonard. "Gender Differences in Competition: Evidence from a Matrilineal and a Patriarchal Society." *Econometrica* 77, no. 5 (2009): 1637–1664.

McDougall, Christopher. *Born to Run: A Hidden Tribe, Superathletes, and the Greatest Race the World Has Never See.* New York: Knopf, 2009.

Whipp, Brian, and Susan Ward. "Will Women Soon Outrun Men?" *Nature* 355, no. 25 (1992).

Willard, Frances Elizabeth. *How I Learned to Ride the Bicycle: Reflections of an Influential Century Woman.* Chicago: Fair Oaks Publishing Company, 1991.

CHAPTER 7: WILL YOU BE MY FRIEND?

Cohen, Emma E. A., et al. "Rowers' high: behavioural synchrony is correlated with elevated pain thresholds." *Biology Letters* 6 (2010): 106–108.

http://www.cupcakinwiththecronettes.com/

Krustrup, Peter, and Jens Bangsbo. "Football for Health." *Scandinavian Journal of Medicine and Science in Sports* 20 (2010).

Master, Sarah L., et al. "A Picture's Worth: Partner Photographs Reduce Experimentally Induced Pain," *Proceedings of the National Academy of Sciences* 20, no. 11 (2009): 1316–1318.

Otto, Michael, and Jasper Smits. *Exercise for Mood and Anxiety Disorders.* Oxford: Oxford University Press, 2009.

CHAPTER 8: TOSSING OUR LACE CAPS

Angier, Natalie. Ibid.

Chakravarty, Eliza F., et al. "Reduced Disability and Mortality Among Aging Runners." *Archives of Internal Medicine* 168, no. 15 (2008): 1638–1646.

DeMaio, Marlene, and Everett F. Magann. "Exercise and Pregnancy." *Journal of the American Academy of Orthopedic Surgeons* 17, no. 8 (2009): 504–514.

McFee, Marcia, and Karen Foster. *Spiritual Adventures in the Snow: Skiing & Snowboarding As Renewal for Your Soul.* Woodstock: Skylight Paths Publishing, 2009.

Mercier, Pascal. *Night Train to Lisbon.* New York: Grove Press, 2007.

Millman, Dan. Ibid.

O'Hagan, Anne. "The Athletic Girl." *Munsey Magazine,* Vol XXV (1901).

Acknowledgments

All the women who so generously shared their stories—what a privilege for me to have been the ear. Libby, for pushing me toward the idea, and for reading along the way. My writing group: Anne, Eva, Louise, Ronna, and Susan, for your wise insight and high standards. To my other keen readers, Auditi and Rachel. Lisa, my agent, and Krista, my publisher, for believing in the project. Merrik, my editor, for holding my feet to the fire and reminding me that every word counts. My friends on the roads, on the trails, in the water, and on the snow: Tammy, Shelley, Rachel, Auditi, Jon, and Kristen, whose company is precious. And most of all, David, my true companion and partner, supportive through all.

About the Author

Mina Samuels is a freelance writer and editor, and in a previous incarnation, a litigation lawyer and human rights advocate. In addition to many ghostwriting projects, her previous books include a novel, *The Queen of Cups*, and *The Think Big Manifesto*, coauthored with Michael Port. When she is not writing she might be off doing triathlons, marathons, biking, cross-country skiing, yoga, rock climbing, kayaking, snowshoeing, or hiking in far off places.

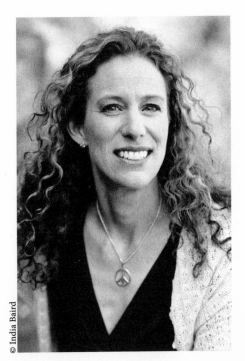

© India Baird

Selected Titles From Seal Press

For more than thirty years, Seal Press has published
groundbreaking books. By women. For women.

No Excuses: 9 Ways Women Can Change How We Think about Power, by Gloria Feldt. $24.95, 978-1-58005-328-0. From the boardroom to the bedroom, public office to personal relationships, feminist icon Gloria Feldt offers women the tools they need to walk through the doors of opportunity and achieve parity with men.

Second Wind: One Woman's Midlife Quest to Run Seven Marathons on Seven Continents, by Cami Ostman. $16.95, 978-1-58005-307-5. The story of an unlikely athlete and an unlikely heroine: Cami Ostman, a woman edging toward midlife who decides to take on the challenge to run seven marathons on seven continents—and finds herself in the process.

A Thousand Sisters: My Journey into the Worst Place on Earth to Be a Woman, by Lisa Shannon, foreword by Zainab Salbi. $24.95, 978-1-58005-296-2. Through her inspiring story of turning what started as a solo 30-mile run to raise money for Congolese women into a national organization, Run for Congo Women, Lisa Shannon sounds a deeply moving call to action for each person to find in them the thing that brings meaning to a wounded world.

Beautiful You: A Daily Guide to Radical Self-Acceptance, by Rosie Molinary. $16.95, 978-1-58005-331-0. A practical, accessible, day-by-day guide to redefining beauty and building lasting self-esteem from body expert Rosie Molinary.

Women Who Run, by Shanti Sosienski. $15.95, 978-1-58005-183-5. An inspirational and informative book profiling twenty very different women and exploring what drives them to run.

The Nonrunner's Marathon Guide for Women: Get Off Your Butt and On with Your Training, by Dawn Dais. $14.95, 978-1-58005-205-4. Cheer on your inner runner with this accessible, funny, and practical guide.

Find Seal Press Online
www.SealPress.com
www.Facebook.com/SealPress
Twitter: @SealPress